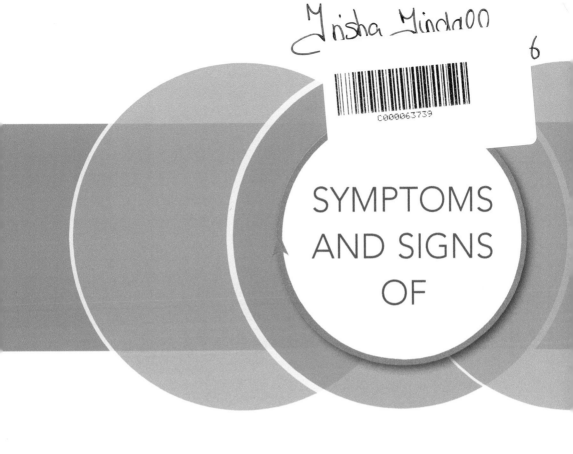

SYMPTOMS AND SIGNS OF

Substance Misuse

THIRD EDITION

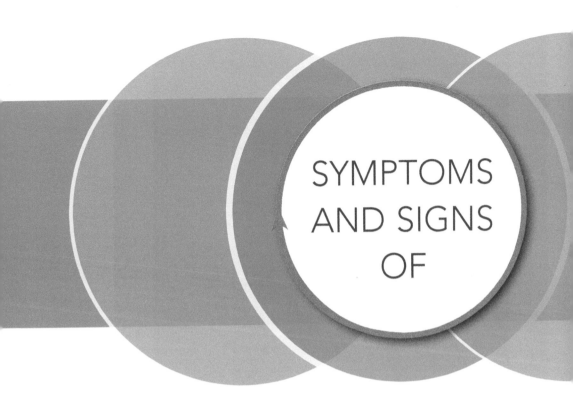

SYMPTOMS AND SIGNS OF

Substance Misuse

THIRD EDITION

Margaret Stark LLM MSc (Med Ed), FFFLM, FACBS, FHEA, FACLM, FRCP, DGM, DMJ, DAB
Adjunct Professor, Central Clinical School, Discipline of Medicine and Sydney Forensic Medicine and Science Network, University of Sydney; Director, Clinical Forensic Medicine Unit, NSW Police Force, Sydney, Australia; Founding Academic Dean, Faculty of Forensic and Legal Medicine, Royal College of Physicians of London, UK

Jason Payne-James LLM, MSc, FFFLM, FFSSoc, FRCS(Ed & Eng), DFM, Mediator
Specialist in Forensic and Legal Medicine; Honorary Senior Lecturer, Cameron Forensic Medical Sciences, Barts and the London Medical and Dental School, London; Director, Forensic Healthcare Services Ltd, Leigh-on-Sea, UK

Michael Scott-Ham BSc, MFSSoc
Committee member of United Kingdom and Ireland Association of Forensic Toxicologists; Member of Society of Forensic Toxicologists; Member of The International Association of Forensic Toxicologists; Senior Associate Member Royal Society of Medicine; Forensic Toxicology Consultant; Director of Principal Forensic Toxicology and Drugs Consultancy Ltd, London; Director of Principal Forensic Services Ltd, London, UK

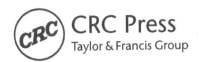

CRC Press
Taylor & Francis Group

CRC Press
Taylor & Francis Group
6000 Broken Sound Parkway NW, Suite 300
Boca Raton, FL 33487-2742

© 2015 by Taylor & Francis Group, LLC
CRC Press is an imprint of Taylor & Francis Group, an Informa business

No claim to original U.S. Government works

Printed on acid-free paper
Version Date: 20140331

International Standard Book Number-13: 978-1-4441-8174-6 (Paperback)

This book contains information obtained from authentic and highly regarded sources. While all reasonable efforts have been made to publish reliab
data and information, neither the author[s] nor the publisher can accept any legal responsibility or liability for any errors or omissions that may
made. The publishers wish to make clear that any views or opinions expressed in this book by individual editors, authors or contributors are person
to them and do not necessarily reflect the views/opinions of the publishers. The information or guidance contained in this book is intended for u
by medical, scientific or health-care professionals and is provided strictly as a supplement to the medical or other professional's own judgement, the
knowledge of the patient's medical history, relevant manufacturer's instructions and the appropriate best practice guidelines. Because of the rap
advances in medical science, any information or advice on dosages, procedures or diagnoses should be independently verified. The reader is strong
urge to consult the relevant national drug formulary and the drug companies' printed instructions, and their websites, before administering any
the drugs recommended in this book. This book does not indicate whether a particular treatment is appropriate or suitable for a particular individua
Ultimately it is the sole responsibility of the medical professional to make his or her own professional judgements, so as to advise and treat patien
appropriately. The authors and publishers have also attempted to trace the copyright holders of all material reproduced in this publication and apol
gize to copyright holders if permission to publish in this form has not been obtained. If any copyright material has not been acknowledged please wri
and let us know so we may rectify in any future reprint.

Library of Congress Cataloging-in-Publication Data

Stark, Margaret, author.
  Symptoms and signs of substance misuse / Margaret Stark, Jason Payne-James, Michael Scott-Ham. -- Third edition.
  p. ; cm.
  Includes bibliographical references and index.
  Summary: "INTRODUCTION Misuse of both illicit and licit drugs is widespread on a global and massive scale. The term
substance misuse is a general term to describe the misuse of drugs. All drugs (those legally obtained or prescribed and those
illegally supplied) including alcohol and tobacco have the potential for being misused. Individuals may use drugs occasionally
(so-called 'recreational' use), for example at weekends, or may become addicted to, and dependent upon, certain drugs. Drugs
can affect all aspects of life including home, relationships, school, college, university, employment, sporting and personal
life. The effects of drugs on individuals or institutions are frequently highlighted in news stories, often coated with a veneer
of excitement, daring or glamour. This can be very misleading. Unfortunately, whether drug use is recreational, or results in
dependence or addiction, each drug will have physical or psychological effects, or a combination of both. Some of these effects
may appear positive - e.g. a temporary feeling of well-being and some individuals may be lucky enough to use drugs without
any adverse consequences. However for many drug users, adverse consequences are frequently seen, and such effects may be
prolonged or fatal, may affect the ability to maintain or seek employment, to travel, and may result in a criminal record. The
undesirable and unwanted effects differ from drug to drug. Individuals may describe physical or psychological effects that
they feel or experience - these are 'symptoms', or others may see or observe physical effects - these are 'signs'"--Provided by
publisher.
  ISBN 978-1-4441-8174-6 (paperback : alk. paper)
  I. Payne-James, Jason, author. II. Scott-Ham, Michael, author. III. Title.
  [DNLM: 1. Substance-Related Disorders--diagnosis--Handbooks. 2. Prescription Drug Misuse--Handbooks. 3.
Substance-Related Disorders--therapy--Handbooks. WM 34]
  RC564
  616.86--dc23
                          2014011150

Visit the Taylor & Francis Web site at
http://www.taylorandfrancis.com

and the CRC Press Web site at
http://www.crcpress.com

CONTENTS

PREFACE

Misuse of both illicit and licit drugs is widespread on a global and massive scale. The term 'substance misuse' is a general term to describe the misuse of drugs.

All drugs (those legally obtained or prescribed and those illegally supplied), including alcohol and tobacco, have the potential to be misused. Individuals may use drugs occasionally (so-called 'recreational' use), e.g. at weekends, or may become addicted to, and dependent upon, certain drugs. Drugs can affect all aspects of life including home, relationships, school, college, university, employment, sport and personal life. The effects of drugs on individuals or institutions are frequently highlighted in news stories, often coated with a veneer of excitement, daring or glamour. This can be very misleading.

Unfortunately, whether drug use is recreational, or results in dependence or addiction, each drug will have physical or psychological effects, or a combination of both. Some of these effects may appear positive, e.g. a temporary feeling of wellbeing, and some individuals may be lucky enough to use drugs without any adverse consequences. However, for many drug users, adverse consequences are frequently seen, and such effects may be prolonged or fatal, affect the ability to maintain or seek employment or travel, and result in a criminal record.

The undesirable and unwanted effects differ from drug to drug. Individuals may describe physical or psychological effects that they feel or experience – 'symptoms' – or others may see or observe physical effects – 'signs'. The widespread availability and enormous variety of drugs – many used in combination (polydrug use) – with many different effects can make it difficult to recognise: (1) if drugs are being used or (2), if a drug is being used, what type it is. Increasingly organised crime syndicates are producing new drugs – often inappropriately termed 'legal highs' – to try to outwit the legal systems and drug laws. This in itself creates further problems, in that the nature of drugs bought and consumed on the street may be completely unknown to the buyer and vendor, although they may be believed to represent a particular drug group. Medical and scientific knowledge are increasing exponentially but will always remain behind the curve when attempting to identify and categorise adverse effects.

This book is aimed at providing concise and readily accessible facts about the known possible symptoms and signs associated with the most commonly misused and available drug groups to help healthcare professionals, employers, police, parents, teachers, partners or friends to identify whether drugs are being misused. The book also summarises the different types of drugs, how they produce their effect, and methods of treatment or management.

The range and mix of drugs mean that few signs and symptoms are diagnostic of a particular drug, and if drug use is suspected further specialist help should be sought from those experienced in the assessment and management of substance misuse. Perhaps the most important guidance is that if a friend or relative's behaviour and demeanour appear to have undergone a change, it is important to at least question whether use of drugs, of some type and in some form or other, may be a contributory factor. As a general rule doctors and other healthcare professionals should consider it appropriate to always ask direct questions about possible drug usage of anyone they are assessing, in the same way as the use of alcohol or cigarettes would be explored.

The legal issues in this book are placed primarily in the context of current law in England and Wales. The medical and clinical principles referred to are similar throughout the world.

As many new drugs are being encountered on a very frequent basis, legislators are reviewing controls regularly and the status of drugs in the book may have changed since publication. Consequently a link to the UK's Home Office website, which details changes to legislation, is included.

For those wishing to explore some of these issues further, this edition includes further reading that the authors believe are key publications and links to sources of information and specific interest.

AUTHOR BIOGRAPHIES

Margaret Stark

Margaret Stark is the Director of the Clinical Forensic Medicine Unit for the NSW Police Force (since May 2011). In June 2012 she was made an adjunct professor in the Faculty of Medicine of the University of Sydney. Margaret qualified as a doctor in 1981 and is a vocationally trained general practitioner. She completed a Master of Law at the University of Wales in 1996.

Previously, she worked with the Metropolitan Police Service for 22 years as a forensic physician and was the first medical director of the Forensic Healthcare Service from 2010 to 2011. As a forensic physician she has expertise in the assessment of detainees in police custody, including providing primary and emergency care, the management and treatment of substance misuse and mental health problems, and the forensic assessment of detainees, where appropriate. She has extensive experience in writing reports for court and giving evidence as an expert witness.

She was President of the Association of Forensic Physicians from 2002 to 2004 and instrumental in the establishment of the Faculty of Forensic and Legal Medicine of the Royal College of Physicians of London. She was the Founding Academic Dean from 2006 to 2011, leading the team responsible for the establishment of the faculty membership examination. She was awarded the David Jenkins Professorship in Forensic and Legal Medicine from 2011 to 2012.

Margaret has been involved in training professionals in the field of clinical forensic medicine as an information provider, on-the-job educator, facilitator, assessor, and planner, and completed a Master of Science in Medical Education at University College London in 2010. She has written extensively in the field and edited the textbook *Clinical Forensic Medicine – A physician's guide* as well as contributing 20 chapters to a variety of publications including *Clinical Forensic Medicine, Encyclopedia of Forensic and Legal Medicine* and *Legal and Forensic Medicine*. Over the years she has been involved in a number of qualitative and quantitative research projects resulting in articles published in peer-reviewed journals and research reports.

Jason Payne-James

Jason Payne-James is a forensic physician and specialist in forensic and legal medicine. He qualified in medicine in 1980 at the University of London and undertook additional postgraduate education to higher degree level at Cardiff Law School, the Department of Forensic Medicine and Science at the University of Glasgow and the University of Ulster, Northern Ireland. He is a mediator accredited by the Civil Mediation Council.

Jason is Honorary Senior Lecturer at Cameron Forensic Medical Sciences, Barts and the London Medical and Dental School, UK. He is external consultant to the UK National Crime Agency and National Injuries Database. He has been a forensic medical examiner for the Metropolitan Police Service for over two decades. He is Editor-in-Chief of the *Journal of Forensic and Legal Medicine*.

Jason has co-edited, co-authored and contributed to publications including *Encyclopedia of Forensic and Legal Medicine* and *Forensic Medicine: Clinical and pathological aspects*; he is lead author of the 13th edition of *Simpson's Forensic Medicine*, co-authored the *Oxford Handbook of Forensic Medicine* and co-edited *Age Estimation in the Living and Current Practice in Forensic Medicine*.

Michael Scott-Ham

Mike Scott-Ham is a forensic toxicologist with more than 30 years' experience of casework involving drugs and/or alcohol. Before its closure he was the principal scientist for toxicology at the Forensic Science Service (FSS) and has subsequently formed the Principal Forensic Services with ex-colleagues to deliver forensic services to a wider audience. He has also formed the Principal Forensic Toxicology and Drugs Consultancy.

Mike has participated nationally and internationally in promoting best practice and presenting scientific papers; he has worked on complex and high-profile police casework and given evidence at court as an expert witness on very many occasions.

He joined the Metropolitan Police Forensic Science Laboratory in 1978 and his casework experience includes several thousand cases covering all aspects of forensic toxicology such as Road Traffic Act alcohol and drugs cases, alcohol technical defence, criminal toxicology including so-called 'date rapes', murders and poisonings, and also coroners' toxicology. He was also an authorised analyst for the Home Office Road Traffic Act until FSS closure.

Mike is a committee member of the UK and Ireland Association of Forensic Toxicologists, a member of the Society of Forensic Toxicologists, the International Association of Forensic Toxicologists, LTG (formerly London Toxicology Group) and the European Workplace Drug Testing Society, and a senior associate member of the Royal Society of Medicine.

Mike has co-authored some high-profile papers including 'Toxicological findings in cases of alleged drug-facilitated sexual assault in the United Kingdom over a 3-year period' and another related paper 'A study of blood and urine alcohol concentrations in cases of alleged drug-facilitated sexual assault in the United Kingdom over a 3-year period', both of which caused considerable interest in scientific circles and the media.

He has also recently co-authored a paper about drugs and driving entitled 'Concentrations of drugs determined in blood samples collected from suspected drugged drivers in England and Wales'. He has reviewed papers for the *Journal of Forensic and Legal Medicine and Science and Justice*.

In April 2013 Mike was appointed to a Home Office expert panel to advise on drugs and driving.

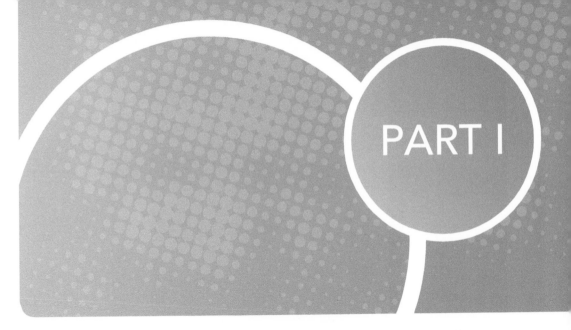

PART I

INTRODUCTION

1 ROUTES OF ADMINISTRATION

Routes of drug administration are the means by which a drug is taken into the body to exert its effect. The speed and amount of effect for a given dose may be modified by the different routes used for the same drug. For medical drugs there are three main routes of drug administration: topical, enteral and parenteral. Topical administration refers to when the drug is applied directly to the area where it is needed. This may be onto a skin surface or onto a cavity lining a structure (e.g. the nose and mouth). The enteral (intestinal) route of drug administration involves the drug being introduced into the intestinal (digestive) tract, which may involve taking the drug orally, infusing it, injecting it via a tube through the nose or mouth, or using suppository or enema-type applications. The third main medical route is parenteral. Parenteral administration covers the various types of injections and infusions (subcutaneous, intravenous and intramuscular).

Illicit drug users may use these, or variations of these, techniques (both intentionally and accidentally). The main route for illicit drugs is orally – by mouth (sometimes placed under the tongue, or rubbed on the gums or mouth lining) and swallowed. Taking drugs by mouth allows the drugs to pass into the stomach. Some preparations are broken down within the stomach to release drug molecules that can then pass into the intestines; this is where most absorption occurs via the intestinal walls through passive diffusion (the site varies from drug to drug) and the drug then enters the bloodstream. Drugs that are typically taken in this way are alcohol, amphetamines, ecstasy, methadone, benzodiazepines, LSD (lysergic acid diethylamide) and magic mushrooms. Swallowing is perceived as a relatively safe way to take some drugs because the substance will be fairly slowly absorbed through the intestinal walls, resulting in effects that are less extreme and therefore less dangerous. Unfortunately this may (particularly in the case of alcohol and methadone) be misleading, causing a delay in the onset of severe intoxication.

The topical route is used for many drugs. Some drugs such as cocaine powder may be applied directly to the gums to achieve a very rapid effect. Direct contact with absorptive surfaces may be achieved via a number of methods: intranasally (or pernasally) inhaled as a pure drug into the nose ('sniffed', 'snorted'), by burning the drug and inhaling the fumes ('chasing', 'chasing the dragon'), or by smoking – mixing the drug with tobacco in a cigarette and inhaling the smoke. Smoking is one of the most common routes of drug administration, and drugs that are typically smoked include tobacco, marijuana, opium, heroin and cocaine. The smoke is drawn into the lungs and rapidly absorbed into the bloodstream. It is one of the fastest ways for someone to experience a high because the chemicals are transferred to the appropriate body receptors in seconds.

Specific side effects of long-term smoking of tobacco, or any drug, may include: a higher chance of developing heart disease, strokes and high blood pressure; mouth, throat and lung cancer; chronic obstructive pulmonary disease (including emphysema and chronic bronchitis); and bacterial pneumonia and other lung infections. An additional risk is that drugs such as cannabis and crack cocaine pose greater risks than tobacco to a smoker primarily because they need to be inhaled in order for a high to be experienced. Not all (tobacco) smokers fully inhale. A variety of everyday objects may be adapted as drug 'pipes'. Figure 1.1 shows an asthma inhaler cover and miniature bottle of alcohol used in this way.

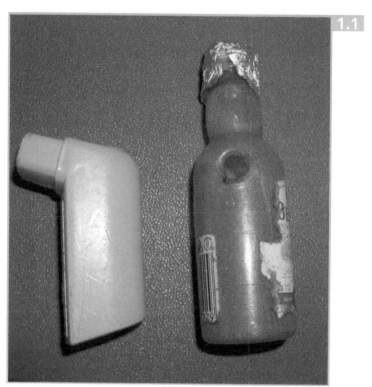

Figure 1.1 **Asthma inhaler cover and miniature bottle of whisky used as a crack pipe.**

The snorting of drugs (also referred to as insufflation) is conducted mostly by users of tobacco, cocaine, heroin, synthetic cathinones such as mephedrone, and ketamine. Much of the snorted substance will enter the bloodstream via the mucous membrane in the nose. In general, the high is experienced within about 15 minutes of snorting. There are several health risks associated with this method, perhaps the most widely known being that drugs such as cocaine have the potential to irreparably damage the lining of the nostrils, damage the nasal cavity, and destroy the nasal septum, the wall of cartilage between the two nostrils. This can lead to quite dramatic disfigurement and has received wide publicity when experienced by well-known celebrities. Sharing implements (e.g. straws, bank notes) to snort drugs has the potential for transmission of diseases such as hepatitis C and HIV.

A number of parenteral routes are used: intravenous ('mainlining', 'fixing') by injecting a liquid form or solution of the drug into a vein; subcutaneous ('skin-popping') by njecting into the tissue just below the skin; or intramuscular by injecting through skin and subcutaneous tissues into the muscle. Using needles is a popular method of drug administration for many opiate users because the full effects of the 'hit' are felt almost immediately, typically within a few seconds. It delivers more of the drug directly to the brain. Injecting illicit substances is one of the more dangerous routes of administration because contaminants (of which most drugs have many) that would not have entered the circulation via enteral or topical routes can enter unchallenged. This increases the chance of infection from contaminated needles or drugs, inflammation and scarring of the veins, and vascular damage at the injection site; the last can lead to haemorrhaging, distal ischaemia, gangrene, endarteritis and thrombosis.

In a small proportion of cases vaginal and rectal administration – placement of the drug directly into the vagina or rectum – is used; in these cases the drug may be absorbed rapidly across the mucosal lining.

Accidental intake occurs, for example, when drugs have been swallowed in packages, in an attempt either to conceal drugs ('swallowers') or to smuggle drugs ('stuffers', 'mules', 'body packers'), and leakage of the contents of such packages – even in small quantities – can be fatal (see Chapter 5 – suspected internal drug traffickers or SIDTs).

Drugs may be presented in many different ways, often as 'wraps' or 'bags' contained in paper, foil or plastic film (Figure 1.2).

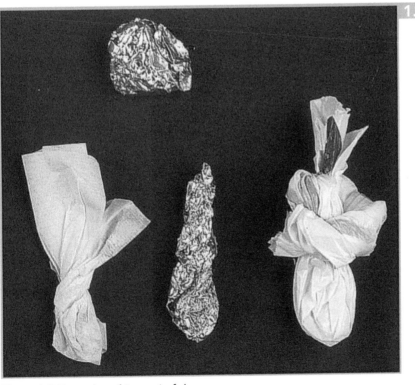

Figure 1.2 **Examples of 'wraps' of drugs.**

2 HARM REDUCTION AND MINIMISATION

For many individuals who misuse drugs, the total avoidance of the drug is not a choice. It is therefore unrealistic to believe that substance misuse will not occur. It is now recognised that, for those individuals who will continue to use drugs, it is desirable to try to reduce the amount of harm that may ensue to both the individual and the community. This approach has been termed either 'harm reduction' or 'harm minimisation'. The first term is more frequently used.

Harm reduction is a term that defines policies, programmes, services and actions that are intended to reduce the health, social and economic harm to individuals, communities and society associated with the use of drugs.

Certain principles of harm reduction have been identified as outlined in Box 2.1.

Box 2.1 Harm Reduction: Concepts and Practice: A policy discussion paper

- Harm reduction is pragmatic and accepts that the use of drugs is a common and enduring feature of human experience.
- Harm reduction acknowledges that, although carrying risks, drug use provides the user with benefits that must be taken into account if responses to drug use are to be effective.
- Harm reduction recognises that containment and reduction of drug-related harm is a more feasible option than efforts to eliminate drug use entirely.
- Harm reduction prioritises goals: harm reduction responses to drug use incorporate the notion of a hierarchy of goals, with the immediate focus on proactively engaging individuals, and targeting groups and communities to address their most compelling needs through the provision of accessible and user-friendly services. Achieving the most immediate realistic goals is viewed as an essential first step toward risk-free use or, if appropriate, abstinence.
- Harm reduction has humanist values: the drug user's decision to use drugs is accepted as fact. No moral judgement is made either to condemn or to support use of drugs. The dignity and rights of the drug user are respected, and services endeavour to be 'user friendly' in the way in which they operate.
- Harm-reduction approaches also recognise that, for many, dependent drug use is a long-term feature of their lives and responses to drug use have to accept this.
- Harm reduction focuses on risks and harms, on the basis that, by providing responses that reduce risk, harm can be reduced or avoided. The focus of risk reduction interventions is usually the drug-taking behaviour of the drug user.
- Harm reduction recognises that people's ability to change behaviour is also influenced by the norms held in common by drug users and by the attitudes and views of the wider community.
- Harm-reduction interventions may therefore target individuals, communities and the wider society.
- Harm reduction does not focus on abstinence: although harm reduction supports those who seek to moderate or reduce their drug use, it neither excludes nor presumes a treatment goal of abstinence.

(Continued)

Box 2.1 *(Continued)*

- Harm-reduction approaches recognise that short-term, abstinence-orientated treatments have low success rates and, for opiate users, high post-treatment overdose rates.
- Harm reduction seeks to maximise the range of intervention options that are available, and engages in a process of identifying, measuring and assessing the relative importance of drug-related harms, and balancing costs and benefits in trying to reduce them.

Adapted from *Harm Reduction: Concepts and Practice*. A policy discussion paper. Canadian Centre on Substance Abuse (CCSA) National Working Group on Policy, 1996.

Key features are the focus on the prevention of harm, rather than on the prevention of drug use itself. The appearance of HIV/AIDS and its link with injecting drug users were key drivers in the development of harm-reduction approaches, which are based on the recognition that many people throughout the world continue to use psychoactive drugs despite (or perhaps because of) the attempts of many governments to fight so-called 'wars on drugs'. Harm reduction recognises that many users of drugs are unable or unwilling to stop using drugs at any given time. Access to treatment would seem to be essential for people with drug problems, but many people with drug problems are unable or unwilling to seek treatment. In many cases this may be due to lack of availability of appropriate facilities as a result of inadequate government funding.

Harm reduction targets the causes of risks and harms. This will, in the first instance, require an understanding of what those potential harms are: (1) in a generic sense (e.g. related to modes of intake) and (2) in a drug-specific sense. The identification of specific harm, its causes and decisions about appropriate interventions require proper assessment of the problem and the actions needed. The tailoring of harm-reduction interventions to address the specific risks and harms must also take into account factors that may render people who use drugs particularly vulnerable, such as age, gender and detention.

Harm-reduction approaches must be practical, feasible, effective, safe and cost-effective. There must be an element of compassion and the stigmatisation of people who use drugs should be avoided. The use of emotive or derogatory terms such as 'drug abusers' or 'junkies' marginalises and creates barriers, meaning that benefits may be lost.

Common examples of harm to the individual user include the development of hepatitis or HIV infection secondary to the sharing of non-sterile needles and syringes to inject drugs. Accidental needle-stick injury from discarded injection paraphernalia may also harm non-users. The provision of needle and syringe exchange centres in the community can reduce this risk. Hepatitis B immunisation programmes for intravenous drug misusers can reduce the risk of infection to the individual by reducing the incidence in the drug-using cohort, and may indirectly benefit the community by reducing costs for hospital care.

3 DRUGS, STATUTES AND LEGAL REQUIREMENTS

This section mainly refers to legislation in England and Wales (www.legislation.gov.uk). Those outside this jurisdiction should acquaint themselves with the relevant laws relating to drugs and drug use. Drugs (both prescribed and non-prescribed) are subject to certain legal controls. Import and export of drugs controlled under the Acts are within the jurisdiction of Her Majesty's Revenue and Customs.

Customs and excise management act 1979

Together with the Misuse of Drugs Act (see below) the Customs and Excise Act penalises unauthorised import or export of controlled drugs.

Misuse of drugs act 1971

This Act provides the legal framework for the control of drugs dividing drugs into three classes – A, B and C (Table 3.1) – and also states that it is an offence to:

- possess a controlled substance unlawfully
- possess a controlled substance with intent to supply it
- supply or offer to supply a controlled drug
- allow a house, flat or office to be used by people taking drugs.

The advisory council on the misuse of drugs

The Advisory Council on the Misuse of Drugs (ACMD: www.homeoffice.gov.uk/agencies-public-bodies/acmd) is an independent expert body, established under the Act, which advises government on drug-related issues in the UK. Due to the proliferation

Table 3.1 **Misuse of Drugs Act 1971: classification of drugs**

Class A	Heroin, methadone, dipipanone, oxycodone, pethidine, fentanyl Cocaine/crack cocaine Lysergic acid diethylamide (LSD) Methylamphetamine (2007), injectable amphetamines Psilocybin (magic mushrooms in raw form) Ecstasy (MDMA), MDA, MDEA, PMA* Mescaline
Class B	Amphetamines Cannabis (2004) Methylphenidate (Ritalin) Codeine, pholcodine, dihydrocodeine Phenobarbital Pentazocine Mephedrone and related cathinone derivatives (2010) Naphthylpyrovalerone analogues (2010) Ketamine (2014)

(Continued)

Table 3.1 (Continued)

Class C	Benzodiazepines
	γ-Hydroxybutyrate (GHB) (2003)
	γ-Butyrolactone (GBL) (2009)
	Anabolic steroids
	Dextropropoxyphene
	Buprenorphine
	Synthetic cannabinoid receptor agonists such as Spice and other herbal smoking mixes (2009)
	1-Benzylpiperazine (BZP) and related piperazines (2009)
	Oripavine (2009)
	Tramadol (2014)
	Khat (2014)
	Zolpidem (2003)
	Zopiclone (2014)
	Zaleplon (2014)

*MDA, 3,4-methylenedioxyamphetamine; MDEA, 3,4-methylenedioxy-N-ethylamphetamine; MDMA, 3,4-methylenedioxy-N-methylamphetamine; PMA, p-methoxyamphetamine.

of the group of drugs referred to as 'legal highs', the Misuse of Drugs Act 1971 was amended on 15 November 2011 (by the Police Reform and Social Responsibility Act 2011) to enable the Home Secretary to place new psychoactive substances under temporary control by invoking a temporary class drug order (TCDO). In all cases the ACMD will have been consulted and advised that the order should be made as the drug is being, or is likely to be, misused and has, or is capable of, harmful effects. The TCDO lasts for 12 months, providing time for the ACMD to provide full expert advice on a new substance. On 5 April 2012 methoxetamine was controlled as a temporary class drug under the Misuse of Drugs Act.

Recent advice from the ACMD subjects 25I-NBOMe, and 5- and 6-APB and their related substances, including some of their simple derivatives (except esters and/or ethers), to temporary control under the Misuse of Drugs Act 1971 from 10 June 2013 (https://www.gov.uk/government/publications/circular-temporary-class-drug-order-on-nbome-and-benzofuran).

Misuse of drugs regulations 2001

The Misuse of Drugs Regulations divides controlled drugs (CDs) into five schedules (Table 3.2).

Table 3.2 Misuse of Drugs Regulations: schedule of drugs

Schedule 1 Controlled drug (CD) licence	No recognised medical use, e.g. cannabis, LSD, mescaline Production, possession and supply of these drugs are limited to research or other special purposes. Practitioners and pharmacists may not lawfully possess schedule 1 drugs except under licence

Schedule 2 CD	Includes diamorphine (heroin), morphine, remifentanil, pethidine, secobarbital, glutethimide, amphetamine and cocaine. Subject to safe custody requirements requiring storage in a locked receptacle (CD cabinet). A register must be kept and comply with the regulations. The destruction of CDs in schedule 2 must be appropriately authorised and the person witnessing the destruction must be authorised to do so
Schedule 3 CD – no register	Includes barbiturates, buprenorphine, diethylpropion, mazindol, meprobamate, midazolam, pentazocine, phentermine and temazepam. Exempt from safe custody requirements (except temazepam, buprenorphine and diethylpropion)
Schedule 4	Part 1: benzodiazepines (except temazepam, midazolam and zolpidem). Possession is an offence without a prescription. Part 2: androgenic and anabolic steroids, clenbuterol, hCG*, non-hCG, somatotrophin. No restriction on possession if part of a medicinal product
Schedule 5	Includes preparations containing certain controlled drugs, such as codeine or pholcodine, which are exempt from full control when present in low strengths

*hCG, human chorionic gonadotrophin.

Medicines act 1968

This Act regulates, in part, the manufacture, distribution and importation of medicinal products. Medicines are divided into three categories under the Act:

- General sales list (GSL): medicines that can be sold from any premises without supervision or advice from a doctor or pharmacist.
- Pharmacy medicines (PMs): can only be obtained from a pharmacy and are sold under the supervision of a pharmacist.
- Prescription-only medicines (POMs): must be prescribed by a doctor, a dentist or, in exceptional circumstances, another health professional.

Crime and disorder act 1988

This Act introduces enforceable drug treatment and testing orders for people convicted of crimes committed in order to maintain their drug use.

Prescribing drugs

The law determines who can and who cannot lawfully prescribe medicines (www.npc.co.uk). It also allows local arrangements to be developed to administer medicines to certain types of patients, in certain circumstances. There are two different types of prescribers:

1. An *independent prescriber* is someone who is able to prescribe medicines on their own initiative from the *British National Formulary* (BNF). Examples of independent

prescribers are registered medical practitioners (doctors), independent nurse prescribers and independent pharmacist prescribers.

2. A *supplementary prescriber* is able to prescribe medicines in accordance with a clinical management plan. The plan is agreed by the supplementary prescriber, a doctor and the patient.

Medicines can also be given by another professional with the instructions of an independent prescriber or via local arrangements.

A *patient-specific direction* is an instruction given by an independent prescriber to another professional to give a medicine to a specific patient.

A *patient group direction* (PGD) is a written instruction for the supply or administration of medicines to certain groups of patients. The instruction is agreed and signed by a senior doctor and pharmacist, and includes the following information:

- The health professional who can supply or administer the medicine
- The condition(s) included:
  - A description of those patients who should not be treated under the direction
  - A description of circumstances where referral to another professional should be made
  - The drugs included and method of administration.

Paramedics can administer certain named drugs on their own initiative in emergency situations. The legislation is regularly amended to extend or amend the list of drugs that paramedics can administer.

Doctors, registered in the UK with the General Medical Council, can prescribe controlled drugs listed in schedules 2–4, inclusive of the Misuse of Drugs Regulations 2001 under their 'professional competency' afforded to them in Regulation 7(2) of the Misuse of Drugs Regulations 2001, without the need for a Home Office licence.

However, an exception to this rule surrounds the prescription of cocaine, diamorphine and dipipanone for the treatment of addiction. These drugs can be prescribed only under a Home Office Licence issued pursuant to the Misuse of Drugs (Supply to Addicts) Regulations 1997. Licences are issued to individual doctors and individual premises.

A licence may be issued authorising the prescription of single (e.g. diamorphine only) or multiple (e.g. diamorphine and cocaine) drugs. Since April 2011 doctors prescribing at multiple premises have needed to be in possession of a Home Office licence detailing each individual location. Licences are not transferable and a doctor moving to a practice at different premises will need to apply for a new licence.

Handwriting exemptions are no longer required to exempt doctors from having to handwrite their prescriptions, although they will still have to sign and date prescriptions.

In April 2012 amendments to the Misuse of Drugs Regulations were made to allow nurse and pharmacist independent prescribers to prescribe any schedule 2–5 controlled drug within their clinical competence.

Health and safety at work act 1974

The Health and Safety at Work Act 1974 places responsibilities on employers to ensure the health, safety and welfare of their employees as far as is reasonably practical, and employees in turn have a responsibility to take care of their own safety and their fellow employees (www.hse.gov.uk). Clearly the use of drugs or alcohol by employees or knowledge by the employer of such use could mean that either or both are not fulfilling their duties under the Act. There is increasing recognition of this fact and pre-employment screening or workplace testing programmes are becoming more common or actual conditions of employment.

Legally defensible workplace drug testing must ensure that any specimens are collected, analysed and the analytical result correctly interpreted, including where necessary a medical review, and ensuring correct 'chain of custody' procedures. The European Workplace Drug Testing Society has guidelines for specimen collection of urine, oral fluid and/or hair testing (www.ewdts.org/data/uploads/documents/specimen-collection-guidelines_oct11.pdf).

Traffic legislation

Section 5(1)(a) of the Road Traffic Act 1988 (RTA) states that a person commits an offence if he or she drives or attempts to drive a motor vehicle, or is in charge of a motor vehicle on a road or other public place when his or her alcohol level exceeds the limits prescribed below [section 5(1)(b)]:

- 35 micrograms (μg) alcohol in 100 millilitres (mL) of breath
- 80 milligrams per 100 millilitres (mg/100 mL) of blood
- 107 mg/100 mL urine.

The new Section 5 A of the Road Traffic Act creates an offence of Driving, attempting to drive, or being in charge of a motor vehicle with concentration of a specified controlled drug above specified limit. A list of drugs and limits has been published for consultation (March 2014).

Section 4(1) of the Road Traffic Act 1988, as amended by s4 of the Road Traffic Act 1991, states that a person commits an offence if he or she drives or attempts to drive a mechanically propelled vehicle on a road or other public place when unfit through drink or drugs.

Section 4(2) of the Road Traffic Act 1988, as amended by s4 of the Road Traffic Act 1991, states that a person commits an offence if he or she is in charge of a mechanically propelled vehicle on a road or other public place when unfit through drink or drugs.

'Drug' is defined (s11 RTA) as any intoxicant other than alcohol and so includes prescribed medications, 'over-the-counter' (OTC) remedies and illegal substances.

A person is considered unfit to drive if that person's ability to drive is for the time being impaired [s4(5)]. For a successful prosecution, evidence is required of impairment at the time of driving and also that impairment was caused by drugs and not something else, e.g. illness or fatigue.

The Police Reform Act 2002 and the Criminal Justice (Northern Ireland) Order 2005 permit the taking of blood from incapacitated drivers for future consensual testing (section 7A RTA as amended).

The Railways and Transport Safety Act 2003 amended section 6 of the RTA to provide new powers to the police to administer preliminary tests – a preliminary breath test (section 6A), an impairment test to indicate whether a person is unfit to drive due to drink or drugs (section 6B) and a test for the presence of drugs in a person's body (s6C).

Transport and works act 1992

Section 27(1) of the Transport and Works Act 1992 states that it is an offence for any of the following people to carry out their work while unfit through drink or drugs; namely a train or tram driver, guard, conductor or signalman, or anybody who works on a transport system in which he or she can control or affect the movement of a vehicle or works in a maintenance capacity or as a supervisor or lookout for people working in a maintenance capacity.

Under section 27(2) of the same Act it is an offence for these people to carry out their work after having consumed more alcohol than the prescribed limit.

Intoxicating substances [supply] act 1985

This Act applies to England and Wales, and makes it an offence for a person to supply, or to offer to supply, to someone under the age of 18 substances that are not controlled drugs if the supplier knows or has reason to believe that the substance or the fumes from that substance will be used to achieve intoxication.

The Children (Scotland) Act 1995 makes volatile substance abuse grounds for a referral to a Children's Hearing. This Act incorporated the provisions of the Solvent Abuse (Scotland) Act 1983, which was repealed in 1997.

The Cigarette Lighter Refill (Safety) Regulations (1999) apply across the UK, which makes it an offence to sell butane gas lighter refills to a person under the age of 18.

Drugs act 2005

The Drugs Act 2005 amended the Police and Criminal Evidence Act and the Misuse of Drugs Act 1971 to increase the powers of police and the court in relation to drug control. Police are now allowed to test drug offenders on arrest (as opposed to on charging), requiring those testing positive to undergo treatment. It also empowers police to authorise intimate searches, X-rays and ultrasound scans on people suspected of having concealed class A drugs with the intention to supply or export them.

International conventions

The UK is also party to the following international conventions:

- Single Convention on Narcotic Drugs 1961
- Convention on Psychotropic Substances 1971
- Convention against Illicit Traffic in Narcotic Drugs and Psychotropic Substances 1988.

4 THE MEDICAL AND HEALTH COMPLICATIONS OF SUBSTANCE MISUSE

Substance misuse can result in medical and other health complications that may be specific to the particular substance of misuse (see below under specific drug) or generic – in that the complications are caused by the mode of substance misuse. Such complications may be the first indicator of a substance misuse problem in the absence of acute or chronic symptoms and signs of specific drugs.

Acute intoxication with a drug can lead to minor side effects such as vomiting, confusion, drowsiness and fainting, or more serious effects such as seizures, unconsciousness, sepsis and death. With chronic usage physical and psychological health effects may occur.

Drug-related deaths in the UK have been declining in recent years and the most common drugs involved are opioids, namely heroin and methadone, followed by cocaine and ecstasy. Overdoses related to opioid use are mainly characterised by respiratory depression, whereas those due to cocaine are characterised by cardiac-related events such as myocardial infarction or stroke, and ecstasy by hyperthermia or hyponatraemia.

Any known or suspected drug misuser should have a full history and clinical examination at regular intervals to determine the risks or establish the presence of any treatable or new complication. This should be done with the consent of the individual. A comprehensive history should be obtained with regard to past and present substance misuse (Box 4.1).

The physical examination should also establish whether there is clinical evidence the individual is intoxicated or withdrawing from a drug(s) at that time, and identify relevant medical conditions. The physical examination should include an external physical examination of the body – because stigmata of drug misuse such as needle

---

Box 4.1 Information required when assessing past and present drug use

Type(s) of substance(s) used
Form of substance used (e.g. cannabis resin, skunk, weed)
How long each substance has been used
How often each substance has been used – daily vs occasional (recreational usage)
Quantity of each drug taken per day (average day)
Amount spent on drug per day (average day)
Method of administration (noting sites of any injection if used)
The time of the last dose(s) of substances
The amount used in the past 24–48 hours
Prescribed medication, especially opiate substitution treatment (OST)
Use of alcohol and/or tobacco
Use of over-the-counter (OTC) medicines

---

marks and needle tracks may be concealed. Box 4.2 shows key features that may need to be assessed. If there is clear evidence of current intoxication, it is appropriate to document baseline conscious level, using the Glasgow Coma Scale (GCS, although it is important to be aware that the scale is specifically for head injury and not validated for those under the influence of drugs or alcohol – Box 4.3) and other vital signs such as pulse, blood pressure, temperature and respiratory rate. A brief mental state examination

---

Box 4.2 **Examination**

Physical examination

The following baseline assessments are essential for all examinations of those suspected of using drugs

- Conscious level (Glasgow Coma Scale or GCS)
- Blood pressure
- Pulse rate
- Temperature
- Respiratory rate
- Eye examination: pupil size (Figure 4.1)
  - Reaction to light
  - Eye movements (nystagmus)
  - Convergence
  - Conjunctival appearance

Other observations
- Skin colour – pallor/flushed
- Speech – content/articulation
- Presence of needle tracks, other skin stigmata
- Presence of tremor
- Yawning, lacrimation, rhinorrhoea
- Gooseflesh, sweating
- Bowel sounds
- Coordination, Romberg's (balance) test
- Assessment of gait
- Auscultation of the heart and lungs

Brief mental state examination
- Appearance (clothing)
- Behaviour
- Speech (rate and volume)
- Thought disorder (delusions)
- Disordered perceptions (hallucinations, illusions)
- Obsessive–compulsive behaviours
- Mood (euphoric, withdrawn, depressed)
- Biological symptoms (loss of appetite, disturbed sleep pattern)
- Cognitive function (orientation in time place and person, memory, concentration)
- Risk behaviours: harm to self and others

Box 4.3 Glasgow Coma Scale

The Glasgow Coma Scale (GCS) is made up by scoring three components: *eye*, *verbal* and *motor* responses. The three values separately as well as their sum are considered. The lowest possible GCS (the sum) is 3 (deep *coma* or *death*), whereas the highest is 15 (fully awake person).

Best eye response (E) – there are four grades starting with the most severe:

1. No eye opening
2. Eye opening in response to *pain* (patient responds to pressure on the patient's fingernail bed; if this does not elicit a response, *supraorbital* and *sternal* pressure or rub may be used)
3. Eye opening to speech (not to be confused with awakening of a sleeping person; such patients receive a score of 4, not 3)
4. Eyes opening spontaneously

Best verbal response (V) – there are five grades starting with the most severe:

1. No verbal response
2. Incomprehensible sounds (moaning but no words)
3. Inappropriate words (random or exclamatory articulated speech, but no conversational exchange)
4. Confused (the patient responds to questions coherently but there is some disorientation and confusion)
5. Orientated (patients respond coherently and appropriately to questions such as name and age, where they are and why, the year, the month, etc.)

Best motor response (M) – there are six grades starting with the most severe:

1. No motor response
2. Extension to pain (*adduction* of arm, internal rotation of shoulder, *pronation* of forearm, *extension* of wrist – **decerebrate** response)
3. Abnormal flexion to pain (*adduction* of arm, internal rotation of shoulder, *pronation* of forearm, *flexion* of wrist – **decorticate** response)
4. Flexion/Withdrawal to pain (*flexion* of elbow, *supination* of forearm, *flexion* of wrist when supraorbital pressure applied; pulls part of body away when nailbed pinched)
5. Localises to pain (purposeful movements towards painful stimuli, e.g. hand crosses midline and gets above *clavicle* when supraorbital pressure applied)
6. Obeys commands (the patient does simple things as asked)

---

should also be performed. The remainder and extent of the physical examination will be determined on a case-by-case basis.

Habitual smokers of certain drugs develop chronic wheeze, which may be improved by abstinence from the drug or use of bronchodilators. Most individuals who have smoked or chased heroin or crack cocaine will have intermittent wheeze (which may be particularly evident during opiate withdrawal).

Many drugs can be injected and people who inject drugs (PWIDs) are vulnerable to a wide range of viral and bacterial infections. Many of the injection-related complications,

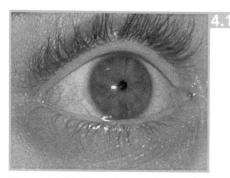 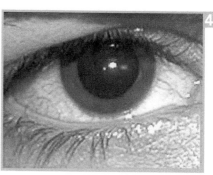

Figure 4.1 (a) Pin-point pupil caused by acute intoxication with heroin. (b) Dilated pupil caused by intoxication with MDMA (as stimulant). (JJ Payne-James)

irrespective of the drug injected, are caused by either sharing (although this has decreased in recent years), or repeated use of non-sterile needles (see Harm reduction and minimisation). In the UK hepatitis B virus infection among PWIDs has declined over the last decade, probably due to the increase in hepatitis B immunisation. Other infections remain common, with 50% of PWIDs infected with hepatitis C virus and 1% with HIV.

Adulterants may be defined as any substance or organism found in illicit drugs at the point of purchase other than the active ingredient. The presence of adulterants can increase the risk of morbidity and mortality. PWIDs often have abscesses, sores or open wounds, which may be infected with *Staphylococcus aureus*, group A streptococci and meticillin-resistant *Staphylococcus aureus* (MRSA). Cases of botulism and tetanus have occurred in PWIDs. In Europe, in 2012, several anthrax cases were recorded from drugs such as heroin contaminated with anthrax spores. Problems can occur whether the drug is injected, smoked or snorted, and users may present with severe soft-tissue infections, sepsis, signs/symptoms of inhalational anthrax or haemorrhagic meningitis.

Particulate contaminants of drugs injected are also a major cause of complications – such contaminants include those that are used to mix or dilute the drug before street sale – and include substances such as washing powder and talcum powder.

Box 4.4 lists the most common medical complications of drug misuse and some of the rarer conditions that should be looked for at an acute assessment.

Box 4.4 **Examples of potential complications of drug misuse**

Vascular

May be short term or longer term:

- Accidental intra-arterial (as opposed to intravenous) injection may cause vascular spasm with ischaemia
- False aneurysm
- Thrombophlebitis
- Thrombosis
- Embolus

Vascular spasm, thrombosis and embolus if severe and untreated can result in gangrene and loss of digits or limbs.

Intravenous injection may be followed by:

- Localised superficial thrombophlebitis
- Deep vein thrombosis
- Pulmonary embolism

Chronic complications include:

- Limb swelling (a mixture of lymphoedema and post-phlebitic changes) (Figure 4.2a)
- Varicose eczema
- Varicose ulcers (Figure 4.2b)

Infective complications of injection

Short-term complications:

- Abscess (Figure 4.3)
- Bacteraemia/septicaemia
- Cellulitis (local – chemical and infective)
- Thrombophlebitis

Longer-term complications:

- Endocarditis (always look for splinter haemorrhages, anaemia)
- Hepatitis:
  - A (several large outbreaks have occurred in intravenous drug users)
  - B (2011 UK 16% of intravenous drug users)
  - C (2011 UK 50% of intravenous drug users)
  - chronic hepatitis: chronic persistent hepatitis (relatively benign) and chronic active hepatitis (progressive); cirrhosis may result and primary hepatocellular carcinoma
  - δ virus infection may be superimposed on hepatitis B virus infection
- Human immunodeficiency virus (HIV) (2011 UK 1% of intravenous drug users)
- Necrotising fasciitis
- Osteomyelitis (haematogenous)
- Respiratory:
  - lung abscess
  - tuberculosis (associated with poor living conditions, malnutrition and immunological suppression)
  - septic arthritis
- Non-infective complications
  - Anaphylaxis
  - Constipation (chronic opiate use)
  - Dental decay (especially with methadone use)
  - Local ulceration (at injection site) (Figure 4.4)
  - Malnutrition
  - Overdose (accidental)
  - Pneumothorax (after forced inhalation of drugs such as cocaine)
  - Pulmonary infarction
  - Respiratory wheeze (non-infective – worse on withdrawal from opiates)

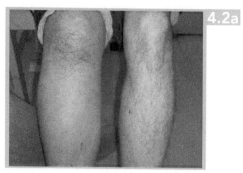
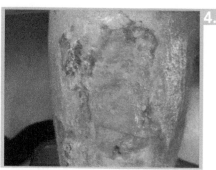

Figure 4.2 (a) Post-phlebitic limb secondary to repeated injection to right femoral vein. (b) Venous ulcer secondary to repeated deep venous thrombosis caused by injection to femoral vein. (JJ Payne-James)

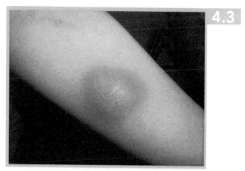

Figure 4.3 Abscess to forearm caused by intravenous drug injection (note gooseflesh caused by associated opiate withdrawal). (JJ Payne-James)

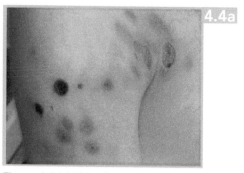
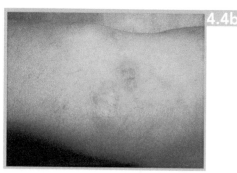

Figure 4.4 (a) Skin ulceration caused by repeated drug injection. (b) Mature scars caused by repeated drug injection. (JJ Payne-James)

There are high rates of co-occurrence of mental disorder and substance misuse disorder. A brief mental state examination should be performed in all suspected cases, considering the appearance, behaviour, speech, presence of thought, perceptual and/or obsessive–compulsive disorders, mood, biological symptoms, cognitive function and risk behaviours (see Box 4.2). Such an assessment of an acutely disturbed patient should differentiate whether the patient has one of the following: a panic reaction; an organic mental state characterised by disorientation in time and space; impaired mental functioning, often with perceptual disturbances such as hallucinations or illusions; or a psychotic illness characterised by delusions and hallucinations in a setting of clear consciousness, often with evidence of thought disorder and lack of insight.

Chronic substance misuse is also associated with psychiatric disorders such as schizophrenia and personality disorders. Depression, bipolar disorder and anxiety disorders, including generalised anxiety, panic and post-traumatic stress disorder (PTSD), are associated with an increased lifetime risk of substance abuse. Traumatic events, such as childhood sexual abuse, may increase an individual's vulnerability and increase the likelihood of misuse of psychoactive substances. Illicit drug users have higher rates of completed and attempted suicide compared with the general population.

Psychiatric comorbidities are particularly common in older people, including intoxication and delirium, withdrawal syndromes, anxiety, depression and cognitive changes/dementia. High rates of mental illness and cognitive disorders result in complex comorbidity in this group, with older people, for example, misusing alcohol with prescribed and over-the-counter (OTC) medication.

Serotonin syndrome results from an excess of serotonin in the central nervous system (CNS), characterised by hyperpyrexia (high body temperature) associated with secondary complications, including rhabdomyolysis (breakdown of skeletal muscle), disseminated intravascular coagulation and acute kidney injury. These toxic effects are more likely with the co-administration of certain drugs, e.g. use of ecstasy with prescribed drugs such as some antidepressants, in particular selective serotonin reuptake inhibitors (SSRIs), e.g. fluoxetine, selective serotonin/noradrenaline reuptake inhibitors (SNRIs), e.g. venlafaxine, or monoamine oxidase inhibitors (MAOIs) such as moclobemide.

To be diagnosed with serotonin syndrome, you must have been taking a serotoninergic drug and have at least three of the following signs or symptoms:

- Agitation
- Diarrhoea
- Heavy sweating not associated with physical activity
- Fever
- Mental status changes such as confusion or hypomania
- Muscle spasms (myoclonus)
- Overactive reflexes (hyperreflexia)
- Shivering
- Tremor
- Uncoordinated movements (ataxia).

Drugs of many kinds, but particularly from the stimulant group, may result in what is loosely termed 'acute behavioural disturbance'. Many healthcare professionals dislike this term; however, for those who work in settings where drugs are used, it is particularly resonant. Drugs – even single or small doses, or combinations of doses – may make individuals behave in a disturbed way. It may be very frightening for the individual and it can also be very frightening for friends, colleagues, law enforcement officers and the general public.

The nature of the behavioural disturbance can be varied and associated with verbal and physical aggression, to the person him- or herself and to others, paranoia and delusions. It may be associated with physical exertion and physiological stress, and put the individual, or others, into potentially dangerous or fatal situations.

The causes of acute behavioural disturbance are not associated just with substance misuse (both intoxication and withdrawal), but also with physical illness (such as after a head injury, hypoglycaemia) and psychiatric conditions (including psychotic and personality disorders). It may be caused by a combination of all of these.

Excited delirium syndrome

Of all the forms of acute behavioural disturbance, the one known as excited delirium syndrome (ExDS) is the most extreme and potentially life threatening. Individuals with ExDS most frequently come to the attention of law enforcement professionals because of the associated violent, agitated and erratic behaviour. Emergency medical services are often called to sedate or transport over-stimulated ExDS individuals after they have been arrested and restrained, or to treat victims of ExDS-associated cardiac arrest.

The concept of excited delirium has become a matter of increasing concern for emergency physicians and other primary care health professionals because many work with policing agencies responsible for policy and procedures, and are used in the field to advise on and manage these patients. The increasing use of new drug groups and an increased awareness of the syndrome means that there is better recognition of possible ExDS. It is important that ExDS is recognised as being the 'cause' of the acute behavioural disorder, because it is essential for the individual to be treated as a 'medical' rather than a 'law enforcement' emergency.

Clinical identification of ExDS is challenging; the spectrum of behaviour and clinical signs overlaps with many other disease presentations. Members of the general public, law enforcement, emergency medical service workers, first responders and even highly trained medical personnel cannot discern the cause of an acute behavioural disturbance by observation alone, nor is it necessary that they do so. All that is required is that they be able to recognise that symptoms consistent with ExDS constitute a medical emergency, leading to the goal of rapid control and initiation of therapeutic interventions. Anyone involved with substance users must be aware that several other specific medical conditions exist that cause altered mental status and may mimic ExDS, including diabetic hypoglycaemia, heat stroke, thyrotoxicosis, serotonin syndrome and neuroleptic malignant syndrome (NMS). Psychiatric issues may also mimic ExDS. Psychotropic drug withdrawal or non-compliance with prescribed medication, substance abuse, many psychiatric conditions, including acute paranoid schizophrenia, bipolar disorder, and even emotional rage from acutely stressful social circumstances may mimic an ExDS-like state. It is not for the general public or the healthcare professional in the field to make the distinction, merely to recognise that in-hospital assessment is required. To this end a card developed by a multidisciplinary panel, reproduced in Figure 4.5, identifies when there is a risk of ExDS.

ExDS Indicators

4.5a

"Excited Delirium Syndrome" is a medical crisis that may be due to a number of underlying conditions. Subjects can demonstrate some or all of the indicators below in law enforcement settings. More indicators will increase the need and urgency for medical attention.

☐ Extremely aggressive or violent behavior
☐ Constant or near constant physical activity
☐ Does not respond to police presence
☐ Attracted to/destructive of glass/reflective
☐ Attracted to bright lights/loud sounds
☐ Naked/inadequately clothed
☐ Attempted "self-cooling" or hot to touch
☐ Rapid breathing
☐ Profuse sweating
☐ Keening (unintelligible animal-like noises)
☐ Insensitive to/extremely tolerant of pain
☐ Excessive strength (out of proportion)
☐ Does not tire despite heavy exertion

Excited Delirium (ExD) Panel Workshop (April 2011), The NIJ Technology Working Group (TWG) on Less-Lethal Devices, The Weapons and Protective Systems Technologies Center

Figure 4.5 **(a)** Excited delirium syndrome (ExDS) indicators.

4.5b
ExDS Response Measures
IDENTIFY
Observe, record, and communicate the indicators related to this syndrome – handle primarily as a medical emergency.
(SEE REVERSE SIDE)
CONTROL
Control and/or restrain subject as soon as possible to reduce risks related to a prolonged struggle.
SEDATE
Administer sedation as soon as possible. Consider calming measures. Remove unnecessary stimuli where possible, including lights/sirens.
TRANSPORT
Take to hospital as soon as possible for full medical assessment and/or treatment.

Figure 4.5 (b) ExDS response measures. (The NIJ Weapons and Protective Systems Technologies Center at The Pennsylvania State University)

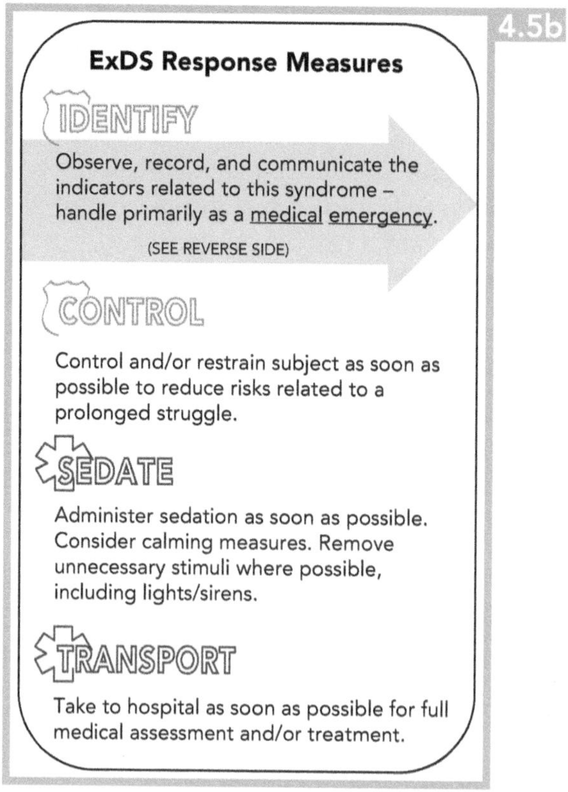

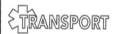

5 SUSPECTED INTERNAL DRUG TRAFFICKERS: DRUG STUFFERS AND MULES

Individuals who swallow drugs to avoid detection by authorities are referred to by a number of names, including 'drug stuffers' or 'contact precipitated concealers'. Drug swallowers tend to ingest small amounts of drugs, e.g. ecstasy, cannabis or cocaine, with low levels of purity often inadequately wrapped in Clingfilm. Such behaviour is not uncommon and may be associated with harmful effects. Police policy has been to treat such detainees as a medical emergency and transfer them immediately to hospital for assessment. Individuals may also place drugs in their vagina and/or rectum, so-called 'body pushers'.

Appropriate training for healthcare professionals and authorities such as police, prison or security staff is essential. There must be a heightened awareness of the possibility of drug ingestion because individuals who are detained by the relevant authorities are unlikely to disclose that they have swallowed illicit substances. At any stage after ingestion a medical emergency may occur, caused by the rupture of a drug package. Signs of intoxication may occur within 6 hours but may be delayed until the packaging has been destroyed and this may take up to 24 hours. Sudden death is a risk from massive overdose of the ingested drug. The risk of harm may also depend on whether the individual is a naïve user or a habituated, with some tolerance to the effects of the drug concealed. Details of the packaging should always be obtained in any assessment of detainees who have swallowed drugs.

Body packers or 'mules' are individuals who deliberately ingest packages of drugs such as cocaine, amphetamine-type stimulants (ATSs) and heroin, often in large quantities, in order to avoid detection by the authorities. There are two distinct types of courier: those who are self-employed and those who are drug mules, the difference centring on the level of organisation and commercial interest in transporting the drug. The drugs are usually of high purity and packaged using machine-manufactured material that does not leak. The packages may be swallowed with anticholinergic drugs to reduce intestinal motility, and prevent the passage of the drugs before the end of the proposed journey.

Body packers should be detained in custody (currently by the UK Border Agency – UKBA) only if constant observation with the custodial early warning system (CEWS) can be provided, supported by rapid access to an emergency department with full resuscitation and acute surgical facilities. Referral to hospital is required 5 days after ingestion if suspected packages have not been passed, because there is a higher risk of intestinal obstruction.

The police have powers to authorise intimate searches, X-rays and ultrasound scans on people suspected of having concealed class A drugs with the intent to supply and export them. The UKBA have similar powers to the police to authorise intimate searches but have no powers to authorise forensic imaging. Healthcare professionals will not perform intimate searches for drugs without the consent of the individual and informed consent is also required for imaging.

Plain radiography of the chest and abdomen, ultrasound and computed tomography (CT) may help with body packers, in the initial detection of drug packages in an asymptomatic individual or in the investigation of a symptomatic individual, but they will be of limited use in the management of drug stuffers and pushers. Any such test may be performed only with the consent of the individual.

Urine analysis may help because, when positive, this may suggest that an individual has used the drugs in the previous few days or that a package is leaking. Alternatively, a positive result may result from the external contamination of packages. Practitioners need to be aware of the limitations of any tests used.

6 SUBSTANCE DETECTION

There are many reasons for testing for drug use, including management and healthcare of individuals, to help control drug misuse by medical professionals including occupational health teams, general practitioners, drug clinics and, increasingly, employers. Such testing requires consideration, including a range of ethical, moral and statutory issues. Other testing may be required for numerous police investigations of drug-facilitated crime including drugs and driving, sexual assault (including 'date-rape', properly referred to as drug-facilitated sexual assault – DFSA), murders, suspicious deaths and poisonings. A coroner, when carrying out a death investigation, may need to know whether an individual has died through ingestion of a drug, or whether a drug played any other role in the death. Family courts may be interested in drug use by parties in care proceedings. Prior drug use by parties involved in insurance claims, e.g. motor vehicle crashes, may be relevant.

One of the most important factors to consider is to ensure that the medium being tested, and the analytical technique used, is fit for purpose. All drugs will be metabolised to some extent and it is essential to test for the correct compound, e.g. there is little point in analysing for a parent drug when it is very quickly, or completely, metabolised.

Different techniques have different limits of detection (the lowest concentration of drug that is reliably detectable), and it can be misleading, if not potentially dangerous, to use an inappropriate technique that does not have sufficient sensitivity to detect the compound of interest.

Required limits of detection for compounds in a workplace drug-testing (WDT) scenario are much higher than are required in forensic casework and to use WDT methods, with their associated sensitivities, for forensic detection would result in significant findings being missed in many cases.

It is also important to consider the difference between qualitative and quantitative/ confirmatory analytical methods. The former are generally used to screen samples for the presence or absence of compounds, often drug groups that are chemically similar, but a positive result is not conclusive proof of the presence of an analyte. The latter are used to confirm the presence of the compound and measure the amount present, when required. There will be differences between laboratories in methods employed, limits of detection and the amount of information supplied in the analytical report/certificate, all of which needs to be taken into consideration when assessing the result.

Screening methods frequently employ immunoassay techniques although, increasingly, high pressure liquid chromatography (HPLC), coupled with mass spectrometry, is used for screening (LC-MS). The latter method may be targeted, i.e. screening for a list of named compounds, or a so-called general unknown screening can be used in which all compounds detectable by the method will be looked for. In recent years it has become increasingly challenging to be able to detect drugs of abuse with the widespread use of many new designer drugs, commonly known as novel psychoactive substances (NPSs), most of which have been synthesised illicitly and for which no certified reference materials (CRMs) are available to use as standards during analysis. In this ever-changing marketplace, new drugs are being encountered on a weekly basis. If there is a requirement to detect all of these compounds, accurate mass LC-MS is an analytical must.

Quantitative and confirmatory techniques almost all employ mass spectrometry, often with gas chromatographic separation but, increasingly, with HPLC separation. Although many NPSs may be detected using accurate mass screening methods, it is not possible to confirm the compound's presence, or measure the concentration present in a biological fluid, without a CRM. Although many compounds will have a specific accurate mass, and therefore potentially be identifiable, the situation is confused by an increasing number of compounds being chemically very similar to others, some merely being positional isomers of another compound, thereby sharing the same molecular formula. Consequently such compounds may not be separable from others using certain MS techniques. Care should thus be taken in interpreting results.

Samples available for analysis include traditional samples such as urine and blood, but other samples are finding increasing applications, including hair and oral fluid. Blood typically offers a window of detection of up to 12–24 hours, with urine offering a longer window of up to 48 hours, but both being dependent on the pharmacokinetics of the drug in question. Oral fluid detection times are similar to those for blood whereas hair may offer a very much longer window of detection, measured in months or even years if the hair length is sufficient.

In some situations blood offers the advantage of possibly providing an interpretation in answer to questions such as how much drug has been taken and when, whereas urine is less open to interpretation. Oral fluid potentially offers an interpretation similar to blood but paucity of data currently precludes detailed interpretation for most drugs.

Hair analysis may offer some limited interpretation if carried out in an appropriate manner; e.g. if analysed segmentally, it may be possible to give an indication of whether a drug has been taken chronically or acutely, which may be relevant in forensic casework, but also in assessing possible drug tolerance in other situations. If no segmental analysis is performed, the only question that can be answered is whether the drug has been taken, assuming that the sensitivity of the method used was appropriate.

Chain-of-custody procedures and measures to prevent sample contamination should be followed in all instances; failure to do so may result in the analyses not being admissible as evidence. Appropriate validated, quality-controlled sampling kits must be used.

Table 6.1 provides some characteristics of common drugs.

Table 6.1 Characteristics of some common drugs

Drug	Half-life (h)[a]	Typical blood concentration (mg/L)	Major metabolites (pharmacologically active or inactive)
Amphetamine	7–34	0.02–0.20	Benzoic acid, hippuric acid (both inactive)
Cannabis (THC)	20–57 (infrequent users) 3–13 days (frequent users)	0.001–0.010 (THC) 0.001–0.050 (carboxy-THC)	Hydroxy-THC (active) Carboxy-THC (inactive)
Cocaine	0.7–1.5	0.05–0.30 (cocaine) 0.1–1.0 (benzoylecgonine)	Benzoylecgonine, methylecgonine (both inactive)
Diamorphine (heroin)	0.03–0.1 (diamorphine) 0.1–0.4 (6-MAM) 2–3 (morphine)	Diamorphine ND 0.01–0.10 (6-MAM) 0.01–0.10 (morphine) 0.1–0.5 (morphine-3-glucuronide)	6-Monoacetylmorphine (6-MAM), morphine (both active), morphine-3-glucuronide (inactive), morphine-6-glucuronide (active)
Methadone	15–55	0.03–0.30	EDDP, EMDP (both inactive)
Diazepam	21–37	0.05–2.00 (diazepam) 0.1–3.0 (desmethyldiazepam)	Desmethyldiazepam, temazepam, oxazepam (all active)
Methylenedioxy-metamphetamine (MDMA)	5–9	0.10–0.35	Methylenedioxyamphetamine (MDA, active)
γ-Hydroxybutyrate (GHB)	0.3–1	80–250	Succinic acid (inactive)

Half-life – $t_{1/2}$: the time taken for a concentration of a drug to decrease to half of the initial concentration.
[a]From Baselt RC. Disposition of Toxic Drugs and Chemicals in Man, 9th edn. Seal Beach, CA: Biomedical Publications, 2011.
Typical blood concentration: the range of whole blood concentrations likely from a therapeutic or typical abuse dose.
EDDP, 2-ethylidene-1,5-dimethyl-3,3-diphenylpyrrolidine; EMDP is 2-ethyl-5-methyl-3,3-diphenylpyrrolidine; THC, tetrahydrocannabinol.
ND, not detected.

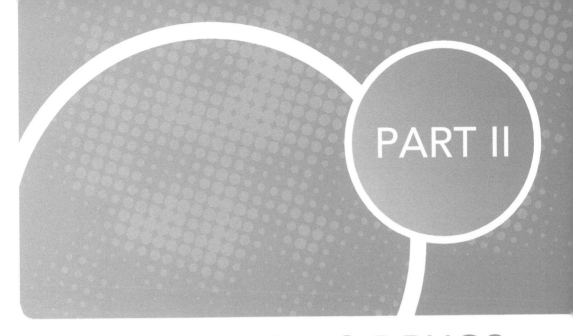

PART II

SPECIFIC DRUGS

ALCOHOL

Principal drugs

Ethanol (ethyl alcohol), methanol (methyl alcohol, wood alcohol, wood spirits). Ethanol and methanol are formulated together as methylated spirits (meths).

Common street names

Booze, hooch, tipple, meths.

Mechanism of action

Ethanol is a central nervous system (CNS) depressant and is absorbed into the bloodstream, mainly via the gastrointestinal tract. Effects commence within 5–10 min. The blood alcohol level peaks within 30–60 min (range 20 min to 3 hours) after last ingestion. The rate of absorption is affected by many factors, including duration of drinking, nature of drink consumed, food (and nature of the food) in the stomach, physiological factors and genetic variation. The peak ethanol concentration reached will depend on factors including gender, weight, height and rate of elimination. The rate of elimination varies within the general population from about 9 mg/100 mL blood per h to 29 mg/100 mL blood per h (median around 19 mg/100 mL per h).

Methanol is extremely toxic to humans, with as little as 30 mL being potentially fatal. In addition to the intoxicating effects it produces as a consequence of being a CNS depressant, similar to ethanol, methanol is metabolised to formic acid which will cause metabolic acidosis.

Medical uses

Ethanol can be used to treat methanol poisoning.

Legal status

The manufacture, sale and purchase of alcoholic beverages are controlled by various licensing regulations. The substance can be bought by adults aged >18 years. Offences include: being drunk in a public place; being drunk and disorderly; being drunk in charge of a child aged <7; or driving or being in charge of a vehicle, while unfit to do so through alcohol (or drugs).

Presentation and methods of administration

Generally it is a liquid that is taken orally. Novel, dangerous methods may sometimes be attempted, including intravenous injection and ocular absorption by, for example, pouring neat vodka into the eye with the head held back.

The concentration of alcohol in drink varies. Average examples are: dark spirits 40%, clear spirits 37.5%, fortified wines such as sherry 18–20%, wine 11–14%, beer 3–6%, lager 4–9%, cider 4–8%.

One unit of alcohol contains 10 mL (8 g) as pure ethanol and is approximately equivalent to half a pint of beer (alcohol by volume 3.5%), 25 mL spirits (alcohol by volume 40%) or one 100 mL glass of wine (alcohol by volume 10%).

Guidelines set by the UK Department of Health recommend a maximum alcohol consumption of 14–21 units/week for females (2–3 units/day) and 21–28 units/week for males (3–4 units/day).

So-called 'binge' drinking is an increasing and substantial problem in the UK, with people going out with the intention of getting very drunk. Such episodes frequently start with 'pre-loading', i.e. drinking cheap alcohol at home before going to pubs, clubs or bars. This is assisted, and one might say encouraged, by the ready availability of cheap alcohol in retail outlets, particularly large supermarket stores. The consumption of numerous 'shots' of alcohol, of various types, leads to rapid alcohol absorption, which is helped by the lack of food consumption, and produces a rapid rise in blood alcohol concentration. A rapid rise in blood alcohol concentration produces a greater degree of intoxication than a slower rate of increase with more noticeable intoxication even at the same blood alcohol concentration, the so-called Mellanby effect.

There have been outbreaks of poisoning where home-made alcohol has been "fortified" by the addition of methanol.

Symptoms and signs

Acute intoxication

Physical: slurred speech, reddened conjunctivae, dilated pupils with a sluggish response to light, lateral and vertical nystagmus, loss of coordination and ataxia, rapid full-bounding pulse, increase in blood pressure and hypoglycaemia.

Psychological: stimulatory effects as a result of disinhibition of the higher brain centres, relief of tension and anxiety, relaxation and aggression may occur.

If alcohol is taken with other depressant drugs, in particular benzodiazepines, opioids or antihistamines, there is an increase in the depressant effects on the CNS with a greater risk of significant intoxication and overdose.

Methanol is poisonous and may cause blindness, coma and death. The effects may be delayed for 12–36 hours as the metabolism is slow. There may be nausea, vomiting, headache and photophobia associated with the metabolic acidosis produced via the production of formic acid.

Chronic

Signs of chronic misuse can include: a bloated, plethoric face, telangiectasia or spider naevi, reddened conjunctivae, smell of stale alcoholic liquor, acne rosacea, palmar erythema, Dupuytren's contracture, gouty tophi, obesity, gynaecomastia, striae, bruising from recurrent falls.

Many major medical complications may occur secondary to excessive alcohol over a period of years including oesophagitis, gastritis, pancreatitis, alcoholic hepatitis and cirrhosis, dementia, encephalopathy, peripheral neuropathy and myopathy, subdural haematomas, hypertension, cardiomyopathy, cardiac dysrhythmias, tuberculosis, gout, osteoporosis, and carcinoma of the oropharynx, oesophagus and liver.

Tolerance to acute intoxication develops with repeated doses and there is a strong physical dependence (see Appendix C for alcohol assessment questionnaires).

Withdrawal

Uncomplicated alcohol withdrawal usually occurs after 24 hours with nausea, vomiting, malaise, weakness, autonomic hyperactivity (hypertension, tachycardia, sweating, anxiety), depressed mood, irritability, transient hallucinations and illusions, headache and insomnia. See Appendix B for a means of quantifying the degree of alcohol withdrawal.

Delirium tremens ('DTs') starts 72–96 hours after the last alcohol ingestion with profound disorientation and confusion, with hallucinations (of any sensory modality), dilated pupils, fever, tachycardia and hypertension. There is a mortality rate of 5% and a low threshold for transfer to hospital should be observed.

Other complications include convulsions, Wernicke's encephalopathy, Korsakoff's psychosis, alcoholic hallucinosis and cardiac dysrhythmias.

Driving

The effects of alcohol on driving ability have been very well studied. The ground-breaking survey in the USA in the 1960s, the so-called 'Grand Rapids' study, demonstrated a twofold increase in the likelihood of being involved in a road traffic collision with a level of 80 mg alcohol/100 mL blood (80 mg%). The likelihood increased rapidly after this concentration and at 160 mg% the likelihood was 25-fold greater. Other studies have shown a fivefold increase in likelihood at 80 mg% and twofold at 50 mg%. Studies such as these have been used to define prescribed limits for national road traffic legislation. The UK still has a prescribed limit of 80 mg% for blood, although most other countries now have 50 mg% or 20 mg%. Some have adopted a zero tolerance approach. Full details of the UK road traffic legislation are detailed in Chapter 3.

Treatment

General: simple intoxication usually requires no treatment.

Observation should be undertaken to ensure that conscious level is not decreasing. In comatose patients general management of respiratory depression and cardiovascular collapse may be required. Treatment of hypoglycaemia may also be required.

Treatment of methanol ingestion includes the cautious administration of ethanol, treatment of acidosis and rehydration.

Withdrawal and rehabilitation

Detoxification can be undertaken with a long-acting benzodiazepine such as chlordiazepoxide or diazepam, and there are a number of different regimens available. Detoxification should be undertaken by those with experience in the management of such patients. Disulfiram (Antabuse) is a deterrent drug, which acts by inhibiting aldehyde dehydrogenase. Unpleasant symptoms occur after a small amount of alcohol such as flushing, headache, palpitations, nausea and vomiting, and with larger doses dysrhythmias, hypertension and collapse. A card should be carried warning of the dangers of administration of alcohol because even a small amount of alcohol, such as that present in certain oral medication or mouth washes, may trigger an adverse reaction. Acamprosate calcium (Campral EC) is recommended for maintaining abstinence (the recommended treatment period is 1 year).

Other or adjunctive therapies and prevention of relapse may be assisted by counselling, intensive psychotherapy, self-help organisations (e.g. Alcoholics Anonymous) or a combination of these.

Further reading

Borkenstein RF, Crowther FR, Shumate RP, et al. The role of the drinking driver in traffic accidents (The Grand Rapids Study). *Blutalkohol* 1974;**11**(suppl 1):1–132.

Jones AW, Andersson L. Influence of age, gender and blood-alcohol concentration on the rate of disappearance rate of alcohol from blood in drinking drivers. *J Forensic Sci* 1996:**41**(6):922–926.

Krüger HP, Kazenwadel J, Volirath M, et al. Grand Rapids effects revisited: accidents, alcohol and risk. In: *Alcohol, Drugs, and Traffic Safety*: proceedings of the 13th International Conference on Alcohol, Drugs and Traffic Safety, Adelaide. Adelaide, Australia: NHMRC Road Accident Research Unit, 1995: 222–30.

Martin CS, Moss HB. Measurement of acute tolerance to alcohol in human subjects. *Alc Clin Exp Res* 1993;**17**:211–16.

AMINOINDANES, INDOLES AND BENZOFURANS

Principal drugs and derivatives

5, 6-Methylenedioxy-2-aminoindane, 5-methoxy-6-methyl-2-aminoindane, 2-aminoindane, 5-iodo-2-aminoindane, 5-(2-aminopropyl)-indole, 5-(2-aminopropyl)-benzofuran, 6-(2-aminopropyl)-benzofuran.

Manufacture

Illicit laboratories.

Common street names

MDAI, MMAI, 2-AI, 5-IAI, 5-API, 5-IT, 5-APB, 6-APB, sparkle, mindy, benzofury.

Mechanism of action

Central nervous system stimulants although less potent than amphetamine and MDMA; may produce hallucinogenic effects. An effective dose of 5-API is 20 mg, around 150-200 mg for MDAI and 30-120 mg for 5- and 6-APB. Half-lives have not been established.

Medical uses

None.

Legal status

Benzofurans are controlled by the Misuse of Drugs Act 1971 class B (from 10 June 2014).

Presentation and methods of administration

Powders, capsules and tablets taken orally or by snorting.

Symptoms and signs

Acute intoxication

Physical: dilated pupils, sweating, high blood pressure, agitation, confusion, hyperthermia.

Psychological: empathogenic effects, euphoria and intensification of sensory experiences have been reported.

Higher doses can result in irrational behaviour, confusion, fear, hallucinations, delusions, paranoia, psychosis. Deaths have been reported.

General/chronic

Unknown.

Driving

All likely to be incompatible with driving a motor vehicle but no known studies.

Treatment

Intoxication: nil – unless complications develop. Then supportive with monitoring of vital signs in hospital setting; intravenous benzodiazepines may be appropriate.

Further reading

Corkery JM, Elliott S, Schifano F et al. MDAI (5,6-methylenedioxy-2-aminoindane; 6,7-dihydro-5H-cyclopental[f][1,3]benzodioxol-6-amine; 'sparkle'; 'mindy') toxicity; a brief overview and update. *Hum Psychopharmacol Clin Exp* 2013;**28**:345-355.

Gallagher CT, Assi S, Stair JL, et al. 5,6-Methylenedioxy-2-aminoindane: from laboratory curiosity to 'legal high'. *Hum Psychopharmacol* 2012;**27**:106–12.

Iversen L, Gibbons S, Treble R, Setola V, Huang XP, Roth BL. Neurochemical profiles of some novel psychoactive substances. *Eur J Pharmacol* 2013;**700**:147–51.

Iversen L, White M, Treble R. Designer psychostimulants: Pharmacology and differences. *Neuropharmacology* 2014;http://dx.doi.org/10.1016/j.neuropharm. 2014.01.15

Jebadurai J, Schifano F, Deluca P. Recreational use of 1-(2-naphthyl)-2-(1-pyrrolidinyl)-1-pentanone hydrochloride (NRG-1), 6-(2-aminopropyl) benzofuran (Benzofury/6-APB) and NRG-2 with review of available evidence-based literature. *Hum Psychopharmacol Clin Exp* 2013;**28**:356-364.

Sainsbury PD, Kicman AT, Archer RP, King LA, Braithwaite RA. Aminoindanes – the next wave of 'legal highs'? *Drug Test Anal* 2011;**3**:479–82.

Seetohul LN, Maskell PD, De Paoli G, et al. Deaths associated with new designer drug 5-IT. *BMJ* 2012;**345**:e5625.

Shulgin AT, Shulgin A. *TiHKAL – The Continuation*. Berkeley, CA: Transform Press, 1997.

Simmler LD, Rickli A, Schramm Y et al. Pharmacological profiles of aminoindanes, piperazines and pipradrol derivatives. *Biochem Pharmacol* 2014;**88**:237-244

AMPHETAMINE-TYPE STIMULANTS

Principal drugs and derivatives

Amphetamine (Benzedrine), dextroamphetamine (Dexedrine), methamphetamine/
metamphetamine/methamfetamine/metamfetamine, *p*-methoxyamphetamine (PMA),
p-methoxymethamphetamine (PMMA), methylphenidate (Ritalin).

Please note that spellings of certain drug names vary from country to country and
anyone using this book should ensure that they are making reference to the appropriate
drug and name within their jurisdiction.

Manufacture

Laboratory based (legal and illegal). Methamphetamine is the most widely manufactured
amphetamine-type stimulant (ATS) worldwide. There are significant public health
risks from illegal production with the potential for environmental fires and accidental
poisoning in clandestine laboratories.

Common street names

Amphetamine: uppers, 'A', speed, whizz, Billy whizz, wake-up, cranks, sulph, hearts,
dex, dexy, dexies (Dexedrine).

Methamphetamine: crystal, ice, glass, meth.

PMA, PMMA: pink ecstasy, death, Dr Death.

Methylphenidate: diet coke, kiddie coke.

Mechanism of action

Central nervous system stimulants (actions resemble those of adrenaline). When
absorbed in the gastrointestinal tract they may have an effect within 20 minutes of
ingestion. There is an immediate effect when injected. The effects last 4–6 h. Mostly
metabolised by the liver. A substantial fraction is excreted unchanged in the urine. The
half-life is 10–30 h.

This group of drugs may be taken orally, nasally, smoked or injected intravenously
(Figure 9.1).

Medical uses

Amphetamine was originally used for weight reduction and as an antidepressant. It
is currently used for the treatment of hyperactivity in children and the treatment of
narcolepsy.

Methylphenidate is used for treatment of attention deficit hyperactivity disorder
(ADHD) and narcolepsy. Methamphetamine, as the l-form, is used in some
formulations of 'Vicks' inhalers.

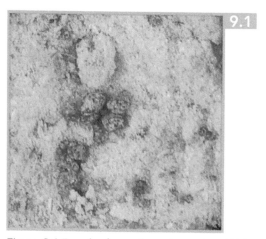

Figure 9.1 **Powder form of amphetamine. (JJ Payne-James)**

Legal status

Amphetamine is a prescription-only medicine controlled under the Misuse of Drugs Act 1971, class B under schedule 2 (amphetamine, dextroamphetamine, methylphenidate). All forms of amphetamine are class A if prepared for injection. Class A: methamphetamine, PMA, PMMA.

Presentation and methods of administration

Amphetamine: tablets, capsules, pale-coloured powders; base is a waxy or oily substance, sometimes with a fishy odour.

Methamphetamine: powder or crystalline substance, also found as tablets; base is a waxy or oily substance, sometimes with a fishy odour.

Methylphenidate: tablets.

PMA, PMMA: pale-coloured powders, tablets, capsules.

Symptoms and signs

Acute intoxication

Physical: low-to-moderate doses (15–30 mg/24 h) result in tachypnoea, tachycardia, hypertension, loss of appetite, dilatation of pupils, brisk reflexes and fine tremor of the limbs. Higher doses will produce a dry mouth, pyrexia, sweating, blurring of vision, dizziness, bruxism, flushing or pallor, cardiac dysrhythmias and loss of coordination. These effects may last for 12 hours or more. Stereotypical behaviour – the repetition of specific acts for hours – has been reported. Pulmonary oedema and myocardial infarction have been documented. Fatalities are rarely reported but predominantly result from convulsions and intracranial haemorrhage.

PMA and PMMA have been reported to be particularly dangerous drugs because the stimulant effects have a slow onset of action such that the user takes more and more ('stacking') and eventually overdoses. Given the low prevalence of the drug, there is a disproportionately high incidence of death.

Psychological: euphoria, feeling of self-confidence, raised self-esteem, lowered anxiety, increased energy, greater concentration, irritability, restlessness. These perceived stimulant effects last for up to 6 hours. Higher doses can result in irrational behaviour, confusion, fear, hallucinations, delusions, paranoia and psychosis. Psychological dependence is observed although physical dependence is not generally considered to occur.

When injected, the user additionally experiences a sensory 'rush' or 'flash', giving almost immediate sensations of enhanced energy and self-confidence and enhanced sexual enjoyment. Users rapidly develop tolerance. The 'high' reported with smoking methamphetamine is supposedly more intense than cocaine.

General/chronic

Longer-term use requires increased dosage levels due to tolerance, with progression to intravenous use. 'Speed runs' describe the repeated use over a period of days. Several grams of amphetamines may be used daily. At the end of the 'run' the user may sleep for several days. Sometimes associated with alcohol consumption; use of cannabis or benzodiazepines may reduce anxiety caused by amphetamines. Amphetamines may be used to reduce the sedative effects of alcohol or heroin.

Physical: long-term use may additionally cause anorexia and weight loss, malnutrition, vomiting, cardiac dysrhythmias, cardiomyopathy, angina, diarrhoea, convulsions, formication, coma and death.

Psychological: in addition to the short-term effects continued amphetamine usage can cause aggression, fatigue, weakness, insomnia, anxiety, depression, suicidal ideation, and episodic, prolonged or occasionally permanent psychosis. Latent schizophrenia may be triggered by moderate use, or even by a single large dose.

Cessation/withdrawal

Users find that cessation can cause anxiety, depression for periods of months, disturbance of sleep patterns, and irritability. Amphetamine psychosis may develop and persist for months or years after cessation.

Driving

The use of stimulant drugs can be associated with risk-taking behaviour whilst the person is experiencing the direct stimulant effects of the drug (e.g. pulling out in front of vehicles where there would normally be considered insufficient time, driving faster than normal).

Conversely it has been reported that acute use of amphetamine in low dosage by tired individuals can produce an improvement in attention for a short period of time, with subsequent improvement in performance of certain tasks compared with the situation in which no amphetamine has been taken. However, the effect is short-lived. Long-distance lorry drivers frequently used the drug in the 1960s and 1970s. US pilots were given low doses (5 mg) when flying long-distance missions in operations 'Desert Shield' and 'Desert Storm' in Kuwait.

It appears that amphetamine, if taken in low dosage and in the absence of other substances, may not significantly impair a person's ability to drive. In higher dosage than that associated with medical usage, the drug can impair driving ability. The after-effects of amphetamine use include poor concentration and coordination as well as drowsiness; none of these is compatible with safe driving.

Drug impairment tests are reported to perform poorly at identifying amphetamine users, with only 5% being correctly identified when low or moderate doses have been taken. Impairment is more obvious at higher doses.

Treatment

Intoxication: nil – unless complications develop. Then supportive with monitoring of vital signs in a hospital setting. Sedation and antihypertensives may be required.

General/chronic: as for intoxication.

Withdrawal: psychological support and counselling.

Further reading

Caldicott DGE, Edwards NA, Kruys A, et al. Dancing with 'death': *p*-methoxyamphetamine overdose and its acute management. *Clin Toxicol* 2003;**41**:143–54.

De laTorre R, Farré M, Navarro M, Pacifici R, Zuccaro P, Pichini S. Clinical pharmacokinetics of amfetamine and related substances. *Clin Pharmacokinet* 2004;**43**:157–85.

Ellinwood EH, Nikaido AM. Stimulant induced impairment: A perspective across dose and duration of use. *Alcohol Drugs Driv* 1987;**3**:19–24.

Emonson L, Vanderbeek RD. The use of amphetamines in US Air Force tactical operations during Desert Shield and Storm. *Aviat Space Environ Med* 1995;**66**:260–3.

Gjerde H, Christophersen AS, Morland J. Amphetamine and drugged driving. *J Traffic Med* 1992;**20**:21–6.

Harris D, Batki SL. Stimulant psychosis: symptom profile and acute clinical course. *Am J Addict* 2000;**9**:28–37.

Hart JB, Wallace J. The adverse effects of amphetamines. *Clin Toxicol* 1975;**8**:179–90.

Hurst PM. Amphetamines and driving. *Alcohol Drugs Driv* 1987;**3**:13–16.

Johansen SS, Hansen AC, Müller IB, et al. Three fatal cases of PMA and PMMA poisoning in Denmark. *J Analyt Toxicol* 2003;**27**:253–6.

Logan BK. Methamphetamine and driving impairment. *J Forensic Sci* 1996;**41**:457–64.

Logan BK. Methamphetamine – effects on human performance and behavior. *Forensic Sci Rev* 2002;**14**:133–51.

Silber BY, Papafotiou K, Croft RJ, et al. An evaluation of the sensitivity of the standardised field sobriety tests to detect the presence of amphetamine. *Psychopharmacology* 2005;**182**:153–9.

Vevelstad M, Öestad EL, Middelkoop G, et al. The PMMA epidemic in Norway: comparison of fatal and non-fatal intoxications. *Forensic Sci Int* 2012;**219**:151–7.

ANABOLIC STEROIDS

Principal drugs

Nandrolone (Deca-Durabolin), testosterone, stanozolol, methandrostenolone (Dianabol), Durabolin, oxymetholone (Anadrol), clenbuterol, trenbolone.

Mechanism of action

Hormones with anabolic and androgenic effects.

Common street names

Gym candy, roids, stackers, weight trainers, gear.

Medical uses

Used in the treatment of persistent anaemia and osteoporosis (although now no longer recommended), for menopausal symptoms, as a supplementary treatment in breast cancer, and to help with protein build-up during or after wasting diseases.

Legal status

Prescription-only medicines controlled under the Misuse of Drugs Act 1971, class C.

Presentation and method of administration

Taken orally and can be injected. May be taken cyclically with different steroids used simultaneously ('stacking'), or use increasing doses of a given drug – 'pyramid'. These drugs are taken by body builders and athletes to enhance their physical appearance.

Symptoms and signs

Physical: hypertrophied muscles, acne, hypertension, abnormal liver function tests, peliosis hepatitis, jaundice, liver tumours, Wilms' tumours, hypertension, reduction of high-density lipoprotein (HDL), increase in low-density lipoprotein (LDL)-cholesterol, thrombosis, reduction in testosterone resulting in a decrease in sperm quality and output, gynaecomastia, hirsutism, deepening of voice, male pattern baldness and decreased breast size in women. There are the usual risks of injection such as HIV, AIDS and hepatitis B.

Psychological: increase in aggression, confusion, sleep disorder, depression, hallucinations, paranoia, delusions of grandeur and reference, and 'roid rage' in which the user becomes very short-tempered and violent.

Driving

No known adverse effects despite reports of steroids producing increased aggression.

Treatment

The drugs should be stopped immediately. Liver function tests usually return to normal. Withdrawal symptoms such as craving, depression and fatigue may ensue. Gynaecomastia may not resolve spontaneously and may require surgical excision for cosmetic reasons. Masculinisation effects on women may not be reversible.

Further reading

Ellingrod VL, Perry PJ, Yates WR, et al. The effects of anabolic steroids on driving performance as assessed by the Iowa driver simulator. *Am J Drug Alcohol Abuse* 1997;**23**:623–36.

Evans NA. Current concepts in anabolic-androgenic steroids. *Am J Sports Med* 2004;**32**:534–42.

Hall RC, Hall RC. Abuse of supraphysiologic doses of anabolic steroids. *South Med J* 2005;**98**:550–5.

Hartgens F, Kuipers H. Effects of androgenic-anabolic steroids in athletes. *Sports Med* 2004;**34**:513–54.

Kouri EM, Lukas SE, Poper HG, et al. Increased aggressive responding in male volunteers following the administration of gradually increasing doses of testosterone cypionate. *Drug Alcohol Depend* 1995;**40**:73–9.

BARBITURATES

Principal drugs

Amylobarbitone (Amytal), pentobarbital/pentobarbitone (Nembutal), quinalbarbitone (Seconal), butobarbitone (Soneryl), phenobarbital/phenobarbitone; Tuinal contains sodium salts of amylobarbitone and quinalbarbitone.

Please note that spellings of certain drug names vary from country to country and anyone using this book should ensure that they are making reference to the appropriate drug and name within their jurisdiction.

Common street names

Downers, barbs, sleepers, rainbows (Tuinal).

Mechanism of action

They are sedative–hypnotic drugs that depress the central nervous system (CNS), potentiating the effects of the inhibitory neurotransmitter γ-aminobutyric acid (GABA).

Medical uses

The intermediate-acting barbiturates should be used only for cases of severe intractable insomnia in patients already taking the drugs. Phenobarbital is used for treatment of all epileptic conditions except typical absence seizures; it is not likely to be misused. Very short-acting barbiturate drugs, such as thiopental/thiopentone, are used in anaesthesia.

Legal status

They are prescription-only medicines controlled under the Misuse of Drugs Act 1971, class B.

Presentation and methods of administration

Oral ingestion as tablets, capsules or elixirs; can be injected as a liquid preparation from an injection vial. Most barbiturates are very rarely encountered since the introduction of benzodiazepines (fewer than 10,000 prescriptions for barbiturates other than phenobarbital in England in 2012). Phenobarbital is still regularly prescribed.

Symptoms and signs

Acute intoxication

Physical: sedation, with increasing doses – slurred speech, loss of coordination, ataxic gait, coma and death. For most of the more powerful barbiturates there is a narrow margin between therapeutic and lethal doses. The risks of complications from injection are increased because they are poorly water soluble.

Psychological: anxiolytic, impairment of memory and cognition.

Chronic

Sedative–hypnotic drugs cause physical and psychological dependence and an abstinence syndrome. Chronic intoxication occurs because there is an upper limit to tolerance with sedative–hypnotic drugs and individuals often increase their regular consumption above this point. There may be nystagmus, difficulty with accommodation and ataxia, and with higher doses drowsiness, coma and death.

Withdrawal starts within 24 hours with anxiety, tremor, insomnia, restlessness and tachycardia; blood pressure, respiration rate and temperature may be slightly raised. Fits may occur, especially with persistent tachycardia (>100 beats/min).

Driving

As most barbiturates produce profound CNS depression, driving while taking the drugs is not recommended. Phenobarbital is unlikely to produce significant adverse effects although normal guidelines relating to epilepsy and driving apply.

Treatment

There is cross-tolerance between the different barbiturates, and therefore any barbiturate can be used to treat the withdrawal syndrome of another. Benzodiazepines may also be used.

If dependent on prescribed drugs, gradual reduction over several weeks or months may be possible. If large doses are used it may be more appropriate that detoxification should be carried out in hospital.

Treatment should be aimed at preventing the medical complications of fits and psychosis with a long-acting benzodiazepine such as diazepam.

Further reading

Betts TA, Clayton AB, Mackay GM. Effects of four commonly used tranquillizers on low-speed driving performance tests. *BMJ* 1972;**4**:580–4.

Brodie MJ, Kwan P. Current position of phenobarbital in epilepsy and its future. *Epilepsia* 2012;**53**(suppl 8):40–6.

Coupey SM. Barbiturates. *Pediatr Rev* 1987;**18**:260–4.

Johns MW. Sleep and hypnotic drugs. *Drugs* 1975;**9**:448–78.

Yeakel JK, Logan BK. Butalbital and driving impairment. *J Forensic Sci* 2013;**58**:941–5.

BENZODIAZEPINES

Principal drugs

Diazepam (Valium), temazepam (Normison), lorazepam (Ativan), oxazepam (Serenid), nitrazepam (Mogadon), chlordiazepoxide (Librium), clonazepam (Rivotril), flunitrazepam (Rohypnol), midazolam (Hypnovel), alprazolam (Xanax), triazolam (Halcion), phenazepam.

Common street names

All: benzos, nerve pills.

Diazepam: (Figure 12.1) vallies, blues, yellows.

Temazepam: jellies, eggs, temazzies.

Nitrazepam: moggies.

Chlordiazepoxide: tranxies.

Flunitrazepam: roofies.

Alprazolam: Upjohns.

Phenazepam: Russian Valium.

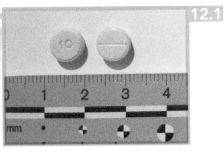

Figure 12.1 **A 10 mg tablet of diazepam.** (JJ Payne-James)

Mechanism of action

These sedative–hypnotic drugs depress the central nervous system (CNS). The benzodiazepine group of drugs produces their pharmacological effects by enhancing λ-aminobutyric acid (GABA) transmission; consequently abrupt cessation of the drugs will result in a reduction in GABA function. GABA is an inhibitory neurotransmitter.

Benzodiazepines (BZs) are classified as very short acting (e.g. midazolam half-life of 2.5 h), short acting (e.g. temazepam half-life 10–17 h), intermediate acting (e.g. diazepam half-life 30–60 h) and long acting (e.g. flurazepam half-life 50–100 h). Hypnotic benzodiazepines would normally be taken at night before retiring to bed. Others are prescribed according to the condition being treated and may be taken several times a day in divided doses.

Medical uses

Benzodiazepines are used as anxiolytic and sedative drugs. They are also useful for the treatment of muscle spasm (e.g. as adjuncts to analgesia in acute back pain). Some benzodiazepines such as clonazepam may be used in the treatment of epilepsy.

Diazepam and others may be used as a premedication before surgery or other diagnostic procedures.

Many of the benzodiazepines are subject to non-prescription use (abuse), often in higher than recommended dosages. Alprazolam has been encountered in illicit heroin powders; phenazepam, which has a very long half-life, has recently been encountered as an abused drug via internet purchase. New BZs continue to be encountered, including etizolam and pyrazolam. Given their fundamental chemical structure many more are likely to appear.

The British Medical Association and Royal Pharmaceutical Society of Great Britain in the UK (*British National Formulary*, www.bnf.org accessed 5 June 2013) have issued advice on the prescribing of these drugs:

1. Benzodiazepines are indicated for the short-term relief (2–4 weeks only) of anxiety that is severe, disabling or causing the patient unacceptable distress, occurring alone or in association with insomnia or short-term psychosomatic, organic or psychotic illness.
2. The use of benzodiazepines to treat short-term 'mild' anxiety is inappropriate and unsuitable.
3. Benzodiazepines should be used to treat insomnia only when it is severe, disabling or subjecting the individual to extreme distress.

Legal status

BZs are prescription-only medicines controlled under the Misuse of Drugs Act, class C and under the Misuse of Drugs Regulations 1985, schedule 4 (except temazepam and flunitrazepam, which are in schedule 3, making it an offence to possess the drug without a prescription).

The product licence for triazolam was suspended in the UK because of adverse side effects, including a higher incidence of psychiatric disturbances.

Presentation and methods of administration

Tablets, oral and injection solutions; suppositories. Normally taken orally or injected.

Symptoms and signs

Acute intoxication

Physical: dizziness, sedation, loss of coordination, weight gain and sexual dysfunction. High doses (overdose) may result in low blood pressure and coma. Death is unusual with benzodiazepines.

Psychological: relief of anxiety, promotion of relaxation, memory impairment. There may be a 'paradoxical' behavioural response with increased aggression and hostility.

Uncharacteristic events may occur: shoplifting, self-exposure, or uncontrollable emotional responses such as giggling or weeping.

There is a 'hangover' effect even in low dosage. The following day there may be drowsiness, inability to concentrate and impairment of tasks such as driving or operating machinery. Phenazepam may cause extreme sedation for 2–3 days.

Alcohol and benzodiazepines increase each other's actions and marked impairment can occur. The CNS depressant effects of other drugs, including analgesics, antidepressants and antihistamines, may be enhanced.

Chronic

Tolerance develops rapidly to both the sedative and the anxiolytic effects. There is cross-tolerance for the BZs, alcohol and other non-barbiturate hypnotics, including clormethiazole.

Physical and psychological dependence occurs with chronic intoxication in those who regularly take large doses.

Chronic intoxication occurs because there is an upper limit to tolerance to sedative–hypnotic drugs and dependent individuals increase their daily consumption beyond this. The clinical manifestations are not unlike alcohol intoxication, with slurred speech, difficulty in concentration, poor comprehension, memory impairment, emotional liability with irritability and depressed mood.

Withdrawal symptoms occur in 20–40% of long-term users who have received therapeutic doses for 4–6 months. Symptoms may occur within 2–3 days of stopping the short-acting drugs and within 7–10 days of stopping the longer-acting drugs.

The withdrawal syndrome results in: anxiety, sweating, insomnia, headache, tremor, nausea; disordered perceptions including feelings of unreality, abnormal bodily sensations, hypersensitivity to stimuli; psychosis and convulsions.

Driving

Many studies have been undertaken investigating the effects of benzodiazepines on driving. Generally it has been found that, when first taken, or if taken in inappropriate dosage, the effects of benzodiazepine drugs on driving ability can be significant. Reaction times are slowed, visual perception may be impaired and time to process information can be increased, all leading to poor driving. Lack of coordination and slurred speech may be apparent. Tolerance may develop if the drugs are taken daily and thereafter the effects on driving ability may be small.

Treatment

Intoxication: mainly supportive because BZs have a high toxic-therapeutic ratio. Flumazenil is a specific benzodiazepine antagonist that produces rapid reversal of sedation; however, it should not be used in the pre-hospital care environment because of the risk of mixed overdoses with complications such as seizures and dysrhythmias.

Withdrawal: change to a long-acting benzodiazepine such as diazepam and reduce dose over a period of time (see Table 12.1 for dose equivalences). High-dose dependency may require in-patient detoxification. The risk of seizures is greater with high-dose dependency.

Dose equivalence of benzodiazepines: what 5 mg diazepam is equivalent to

Drug	Dose
• Chlordiazepoxide	15 mg
• Loprazolam	500 μg
• Lorazepam	500 μg
• Oxazepam	15 mg
• Temazepam	10 mg
• Nitrazepam	5 mg

Further reading

Barbone F, McMahon AD, Davey PG, et al. Association of road-traffic accidents with benzodiazepine use. *Lancet* 1998;**352**:1331–6.

Berghaus G, Sticht G, Grellner W, Lenz D, Naumann Th, Wiesenmüller S. Meta-analysis of empirical studies concerning the effects of medicines and illegal drugs including pharmacokinetics on safe driving. Driving under the Influence of Drugs, Alcohol and Medicines (DRUID). Brussels, European Commission, Directorate-General for Energy and Transport, 2010.

Driving under the Influence of Drugs, Alcohol and Medicines (DRUID). 6th Framework Programme. Available from: http://www.druid-project.eu/Druid/EN/deliverales-list/downloads/Deliverable_1_1_2_B.pdf?__blob=publicationFile&v=1 (accessed 9 June 2013).

Drummer OH. Benzodiazepines – effects on human performance and behaviour. *Forensic Sci Rev* 2008;**14**:2–14.

Greenblatt DJ. Pharmacology of benzodiazepine hypnotics. *J Clin Psychiatry* 1992;**53**:7–13.

Hojer J, Baehrendtz S, Gustaffson L. Benzodiazepine poisoning: experience of 702 admissions to an intensive care unit during a 14-year period. *J Intern Med* 1989;**226**:117–22.

Kelly E, Darke S, Ross JA. Review of drug use and driving: Epidemiology, impairment, risk factors, and risk perceptions. *Drug Alcohol Rev* 2004;**23**:319–44.

Kurtz SP, Surratt HL, Levi-Minzi MA, et al. Benzodiazepine dependence among multidrug users in the club scene. *Drug Alcohol Depend* 2011;**119**:99–105.

Maskell PD, De Paoli G, Nitin Seetohul L, et al. Phenazepam: the drug that came in from the cold. *J Forensic Legal Med* 2012;**19**:122–5.

Rapoport MJ, Lanctôt KL, Streiner DL, et al. Benzodiazepine use and driving: a meta-analysis. *J Clin Psychiatry* 2009;**70**:663–73.

Smink BE, Lusthof KJ, de Grier JJ, et al. The relation between the blood benzodiazepine concentration and performance in suspected impaired drivers. *J Forensic Legal Med* 2008;**15**:483–8.

Smink BE, Egberts AC, Lusthof KJ, et al. The relationship between benzodiazepine use and traffic accidents: a systematic literature review. *CNS Drugs* 2010;**24**:639–53.

CANNABIS

Principal drugs

Cannabis is the common name for the plant *Cannabis sativa* (Figure 13.1), which contains a large number of active compounds known collectively as cannabinoids, the most important, and active, of which is known as tetrahydrocannabinol (THC). It is a mild sedative, which is used for its euphoric and relaxing properties. It is the most widely misused controlled drug in the UK.

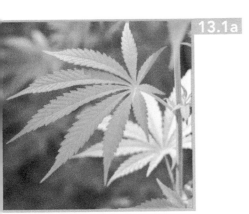 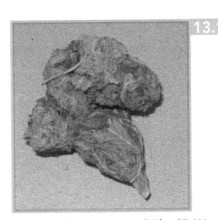

Figure 13.1 **(a)** Cannabis leaf (Shutterstock); **(b)** dried cannabis fruiting material ("bud") (JJ Payne-James).

Manufacture

Most cannabis used these days is in the form of the herbal material, rather than the previously widely used cannabis resin. Most herbal cannabis is now grown within the UK, often in large quantities amounting to commercial production. Such production may use sophisticated growing conditions, which can be on an industrial scale in warehouses, although in recent years converted lofts, garages or other rooms are more frequently encountered. Such outfits will normally use a means of bypassing the electricity meter because they use large amounts of energy. Extraction filters are also often used to remove the characteristic odour. The plants are normally cuttings taken from a mother plant, and are therefore genetically identical and often grown in a fibrous medium without soil (hydroponics).

Common street names

Pot, dope, blow, grass, marijuana, ganja, nabis, weed, hash, hashish, draw, puff, skunk, sinsemilla.

Mechanism of action

THC is absorbed rapidly in the lungs and the plasma concentration peaks quickly, within a few minutes, although peak effects occur later at about 15–30 mins and last for 2–4 h. If ingested orally the onset of action is slower, although the effects last longer perhaps up to 8 h. THC is very fat soluble and rapidly deposited in fatty tissue around the body. Consequently, THC may leak out of fat into the bloodstream over a long period of time after the last use. If a regular, heavy user of the drug abstains for a period, there may still be detectable amounts of THC in the blood for many days and in urine for weeks afterwards.

THC breaks down in the body to THC-COOH (carboxy-THC), which is inactive, via THC-OH (hydroxy-THC), which is pharmacologically active. There are hundreds of other cannabinoids present within the material, including cannabidiol (CBD) and cannabinol (CBN). Home-grown strains of cannabis may contain THC at a concentration in excess of 30% when harvested, although the normal value may be closer to around 10% THC; however, this is still much stronger than foreign imported cannabis which is normally of THC strength 3–4%.

There is increasing evidence that another cannabinoid, CBD, may moderate some of the less pleasant effects of THC. Typical herbal cannabis contains THC and CBD, whereas some of the specially bred varieties, often referred to as 'skunk' on account of the potent odour, may contain THC with only minimal or no CBD. This may account for the increasingly reported adverse effects after heavy cannabis ('skunk') use.

The ninth report of the House of Lords Science and Technology Committee (1998) defined categories of cannabis users:

- A *casual user* may be defined as someone who is an irregular cannabis user, smoking in amounts of up to 1 g at a time but not more than 28 g/year.
- A *regular user* can be defined as smoking 0.5 g/day in three to four joints (i.e. about 150 mg cannabis per cigarette), adding up to about 3.5 g/week.
- A *heavy user* can be defined as smoking more than 3.5 g/day and ≥28 g/week. This group is likely to be more or less permanently intoxicated – 'stoned'.

Medical uses

Cannabis may help symptoms such as muscle spasm in patients with multiple sclerosis and for the nausea and vomiting induced by chemotherapy. Many users claim that it has analgesic properties. In the last 10 years medicinal preparations have been licensed for restricted use in many countries including, for example, the UK and the USA for treating conditions such as mentioned above.

Legal status

Cannabis is a controlled drug under the Misuse of Drugs Act 1971. It is illegal to grow, possess or supply the drug. The Home Office can grant a licence for special purposes such as research. Herbal cannabis (except seeds and stalks), cannabis resin and cannabis oil are classified as class B drugs. THC, when separated, is a class A drug.

Presentation and methods of administration

Forms of cannabis include herbal material, resin and oil. Cannabis resin is a concentrated form of the herbal material, made with those parts of the plant that contain the greatest concentration of the active component; this is preferentially removed and formed into hard blocks. Cannabis oil (hash oil) is a liquid extraction of cannabis evaporated down to increase the concentration of the active component.

The drug is normally used by smoking in the form of a cigarette, commonly referred to as a 'reefer', 'joint' or 'spliff'. However, the drug can also be smoked via a pipe, sometimes an elaborate construction called a 'bong', and is occasionally taken orally in the form of cakes or other fat-containing food, which allows the THC to be extracted (e.g. from chocolate or cookies).

Symptoms and signs

The exact effects of cannabis are reported to depend on the amount used, the social setting, and the user's expectations and previous experience with the drug. Cannabis is usually smoked with effects starting within seconds, peaking between 15 and 30 min, and lasting for 2 h. Occasionally effects may last up to 4 h. However, this will also depend on factors such as the number and depth of inhalations from each 'joint' smoked.

Acute intoxication

Physical: dryness of the mouth, hunger ('munchies'), reddened conjunctivae, increased blood pressure associated with postural hypotension and tachycardia, with slight impairment of psychomotor and cognitive function.

Psychological: a feeling of wellbeing, euphoria, and increased self-confidence, relaxation; perceptions, e.g. smell, taste and hearing may be enhanced. There may be poor concentration, memory impairment, suggestibility and difficulty with tasks requiring manual dexterity. Occasionally anxiety, agitation and paranoia or a toxic psychosis may occur. Flashbacks may occur after the effects of the drugs wear off, more commonly when other drugs such as LSD have been used as well. The effects from the more potent home-grown varieties are likely to be more intense and may last for longer than non-'skunk' varieties.

Chronic

Before the appearance of 'skunk' cannabis there was little clear evidence that cannabis use caused physical or mental health problems in the long term. More recently there have been increasing numbers of mental health problems identified.

Cannabis psychosis may occur after consumption of a large quantity of cannabis or following frequent consumption of high-potency forms of the drug. Confusion occurs suddenly, and is associated with delusions, hallucinations and emotional lability. There may be temporary amnesia with disorientation, depersonalisation and paranoia. There may also be a cannabis-induced functional psychosis, which responds swiftly to antipsychotic medication, but tends to relapse with resumption of cannabis usage.

High-dose chronic use may result in reduced testosterone and sperm count, reduced fertility in women and premature birth, with a corresponding reduction in fetal birthweight.

Gynaecomastia may also occur. There may be an effect on the immune system, making users more susceptible to bacterial infections. There have been suggestions that prolonged use of cannabis may lead to brain damage but there is no conclusive evidence for this. Frequent inhalation of cannabis smoke over a long period may result in respiratory problems such as bronchitis and perhaps lung cancer (although this may relate in part to concurrent tobacco usage).

Tolerance develops rapidly within a few days of regular drug use and decays rapidly when drug use ceases. With very heavy use physical dependence may occur, with a mild abstinence syndrome starting a few hours after stopping the drug and lasting for 4–5 days.

Withdrawal can result in irritability, restlessness, decreased appetite and weight loss.

Driving

Studies have shown that THC impairs driving in a dose-related manner. Maximum impairment after cannabis use is seen around 30–45 min after smoking, with the effects dissipating over the next 2–3 h.

Effects produced by cannabis relevant to driving can include a slowing of decision-making and reaction time, impairment of ability to maintain road positioning, impairment of ability to perform tasks requiring divided attention, impaired peripheral vision, lack of concentration and fatigue. Some drivers may compensate for this by driving more slowly and a not infrequent scenario is for a driver to be brought to the attention of the police by driving very slowly.

Significant impairment of driving performance would not normally be expected to be observed for more than 1–2 h after use. Cannabis use would not normally be expected to be associated with risk-taking activities.

The prevalence of the involvement of cannabis in road traffic collisions and fatalities is unclear, due to the rapid breakdown of THC in the body and its instability in vitro once a blood sample has been taken.

Treatment

There is no specific treatment.

Further reading

Asbridge M, Hayden JA, Cartwright JL. Acute cannabis consumption and motor vehicle collision risk: systematic review of observational studies and meta-analysis. *BMJ* 2012;**344**:e536.

Berghaus G, Sticht G, Grellner W, Lenz D, Naumann Th, Wiesenmüller S. Meta-analysis of empirical studies concerning the effects of medicines and illegal drugs including pharmacokinetics on safe driving. Driving under the Influence of Drugs, Alcohol and Medicines (DRUID). Brussels, European Commission, Directorate-General for Energy and Transport, 2010.

Böcker KBE, Gerritsen J, Hunault CC, Kruidenier M, Mensinga TT, Kenemans JL. Cannabis with high Δ9-THC contents affects perception and visual selective attention. *Pharmacol Biochem Behav* 2010;**96**:67–74.

Bosker WM, Kuypers KP, Theunissen EL, et al. Medicinal Δ(9)-tetrahydrocannabinol (dronabinol) impairs on-the-road driving performance of occasional and heavy cannabis users but is not detected in Standard Field Sobriety Tests. *Addiction* 2012;**107**:1837–44.

Consroe P, Musty R, Rein J, et al. The perceived effects of smoked cannabis on patients with multiple sclerosis. *Eur Neurol* 1997;**38**:44–8.

Driving under the Influence of Drugs, Alcohol and Medicines (DRUID). 6th Framework Programme. Available from: http://www.druid-project.eu/Druid/EN/deliverales-list/downloads/Deliverable_1_1_2_B.pdf?__blob=publicationFile&v=1 (accessed 9 June 2013).

House of Lords. *Cannabis. Science and Technology. Ninth Report*, 1998. (accessed 9 June 2013).

Huestis MA. Cannabis (marijuana) – Effects on human behavior and performance. *Forensic Sci Rev* 2002;**14**:15–60.

Moskowitz H. Marijuana and driving. *Acc Anal Prevent* 1985;**17**:323–45.

Murray JB. Marijuana's effects on human cognitive functions, psychomotor functions, and personality. *J Gen Psychol* 1985;**113**:23–55.

Papafotiou K, Carter JD, Stough C. The relationship between performance on the standardised field sobriety tests, driving performance and the level of delta-9-tetrahydrocannabinol (THC) in blood. *Forensic Sci Int* 2005;**155**:172–8.

Potter DJ, Clark P, Brown MB. Potency of delta (9)-THC and other cannabinoids in cannabis in England in 2005: implications for psychoactivity and pharmacology. *J Forensic Sci* 2008;**53**:90–4.

Thomas H. Psychiatric symptoms in cannabis users. *Br J Psychiatry* 1993;**163**:141–9.

Ward NJ, Dye L. *Cannabis and Driving – a review of the literature and commentary*. UK DETR Road Safety Research Report No.12. London: DETR,1999.

COCAINE

This is an alkaloid derived from the leaves of the coca bush (*Erythroxylon coca*) which grows predominantly in South America but to a lesser extent in Africa, the Far East and India.

Principal drugs and derivatives

Cocaine hydrochloride, cocaine base, crack. A number of synthetic "caines" have appeared for sale via the internet and in headshops. These include dimethocaine and 4-fluorotropacocaine.

Manufacture

It is refined through a number of purification stages in illegal factories from leaves to paste to cocaine hydrochloride.

Common street names

Coke, 'C', charlie, wash, nose-candy, crack, rock, snow, stone, oxi, oxidado. Synthetic "caines" have been referred to by the street names mind melt, amplify, mania and stardust.

Mechanism of action

As a central nervous system (CNS) stimulant cocaine blocks reuptake of dopamine and, to a lesser extent, noradrenaline and serotonin. It is metabolised primarily to benzoylecgonine and ecgonine methyl ester in the liver. Some cocaine (20%) is excreted unchanged in the urine. The half-life of cocaine is 0.7–1.5 h, that of benzoylecgonine 7–8 h. Benzoylecgonine may be detected for several days after last use. The onset of action, half-life and duration of effects depend on the route of administration. When sniffed/snorted, the effects are felt within a few minutes and last up to a maximum of an hour; doses may have to be repeated every 20 min. If smoked or injected the effects are immediate and last 15–30 min.

Cocaine may be subject to repeated use (binging) which can last many hours or even a day or two.

The stimulant effects last longer, but are less intense, and the comedown is somewhat moderated if used together with alcohol. Rebound sedation may be noted due to neurotransmitter depletion.

Medical uses

Cocaine was used as a surface anaesthetic (e.g. in ear/nose/throat surgery) but this is now rare.

Legal status

Cocaine is a prescription-only medicine, class A under schedule 2 of the Misuse of Drugs Act 1971. The synthetic "caines" are currently not subject to control.

Presentation and methods of administration

Ear, nose and throat surgery: as an oromucosal solution (10%) or nasal spray.

Illicit cocaine can be encountered in various forms including:

Coca leaf: normally chewed or made into an infusion ("coca tea") although such use is uncommon outside the countries of origin.

White crystals/powder (cocaine hydrochloride): may be snorted through a straw or rolled-up paper, e.g. bank note in 'lines', or from a small 'coke spoon', or may be injected into veins or applied to mucous membranes (e.g. mouth/rectum/vagina).

'Crack', base, paste: cocaine hydrochloride powder may be basified to produce 'crack' (Figure 14.1), which can be a potent form of cocaine, by mixing it with baking soda and heating. The product is variable in appearance – as white or yellow, small, waxy-looking lumps that may be smoked in cigarettes or pipe; it may also be mixed with heroin and injected ("snowballing" or "speedballing"). Special water pipes are used by some to prevent destruction of the smoked drug by high temperatures. Homemade pipes can be made from a variety of readily available items such as glass or plastic bottles and silver foil.

Synthetic "caines": are normally encountered as white powders and are taken via snorting.

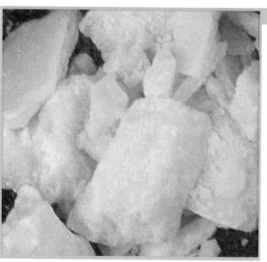

Figure 14.1 **Crack cocaine. (JJ Payne-James)**

Symptoms and signs

Acute intoxication

Physical: the effects are short acting, but dose dependent. The user may experience tachycardia, sweating, significant pupillary dilatation, pyrexia, reduced appetite, reduced need for sleep or formication. It can present as a condition known as 'excited delirium syndrome' (see Chapter 4). Death may occur rapidly secondary to convulsion, intracranial haemorrhage, respiratory arrest or cardiac arrhythmias. The risk of an adverse event is increased if used together with alcohol, resulting in the formation of cocaethylene.

Psychological: euphoria, sensation of increased physical and mental wellbeing; these may be followed by irritability, depression and insomnia; paranoia may develop.

General/chronic

Physical: in addition to the above effects, chest pains and muscle spasms may occur. Impotence and failure of ejaculation have been reported in men, and difficulty in achieving orgasm in women. Rhinorrhoea (runny nose), eczema localised around the nose and nasal septum damage (erosions, necrosis, perforations) with anosmia can develop. Weight loss and malnutrition are common.

Psychological: as for acute intoxication. Tolerance develops. A heavy cocaine user may ingest up to several grams daily. Disturbance of eating and sleeping patterns may occur.

Cessation/withdrawal

It is now generally accepted that physical and marked psychological dependence occurs. This is manifest with muscle pains and tremor, hunger, irritability, depression, fatigue and prolonged sleep episodes, which can last for 24 hours or more. Psychological dependence with craving and intense drug-seeking behaviour occurs. A severe withdrawal syndrome known as 'the crash' occurs.

Driving

The use of stimulant drugs can be associated with risk-taking while the person is experiencing the direct stimulant effects of the drug (e.g. pulling out in front of vehicles when normally there would be insufficient time, driving faster than normal). However, with cocaine these stimulant effects last for only a short period of time, after which the after-effects start. It has been reported that acute (i.e. one-off) use of cocaine by tired individuals can produce an improvement in attention for a short period of time, with subsequent improvement in performance of simple tasks. As the tasks become more complex, however, this improvement may not occur.

The after-effects of cocaine use include poor concentration and coordination as well as drowsiness, all of which are not compatible with safe driving. Lapses of attention and ignoring stimuli such as changing traffic lights have been reported by all users in one study.

Some cocaine users report disturbances in their peripheral vision ('snow lights'), which distracts attention; visual impairment, primarily caused by an increased sensitivity to light, has been reported by many users, presumably due to the pupillary dilatation produced by cocaine.

The studies performed investigating the effects of cocaine on driving have been limited by the dosages permitted because only low-dose studies have been authorised, given the dangers associated with cocaine use.

A study of cocaine-dependent individuals showed a slower reaction time than in non-dependent individuals, which was still evident 3 months after drug cessation.

Drug impairment tests are reported to perform poorly in identifying cocaine users, with almost half of such users performing 'normally' on such tests when prior cocaine use had been established via laboratory testing of urine specimens.

Treatment

Intoxication: nil unless complications develop. Then treatment is supportive with monitoring of vital signs in a hospital setting, using fluids, cooling and sedation as required, together with treatment of complications such as seizures, coronary syndromes and arrhythmias as they occur.

General/chronic: as for intoxication.

Withdrawal

This needs psychological support and counselling, including treatment of depression and sleep disturbance.

Further reading

Andrews P. Cocaethylene toxicity. *J Addict Dis* 1997;**16**:75–84.

Awtry EH, Philippides GJ. Alcoholic and cocaine-associated cardiomyopathies. *Prog Cardiovasc Dis* 2010;**52**:289–99.

Benowitz NL. Clinical pharmacology and toxicology of cocaine. *Pharmacol Toxicol* 1993;**72**:3–12.

Brookoff D, Cook CS, Williams C, et al. Testing reckless drivers for cocaine and marijuana. *N Engl J Med* 1994;**331**:518–22.

Cone EJ. Pharmacokinetics and pharmacodynamics of cocaine. *J Analyt Toxicol* 1995;**19**:459–78.

Ellinwood EH, Nikaido AM. Stimulant induced impairment: a perspective across dose and duration of use. *Alcohol Drugs Driv* 1987;**3**:19–24.

Gawin FH, Kleber HD. Abstinence symptomatology and psychiatric diagnosis in cocaine abusers. *Arch Gen Psychiatry* 1986;**43**:107–13.

Glossop M, Griffiths P, Powis B, et al. Cocaine: patterns of use, route of administration and severity of dependence. *Br J Psychiatry* 1994;**164**:660–4.

Isenschmid DS. Cocaine – effects on human performance and behavior. *Forensic Sci Rev* 2002;**14**:62–100.

McCance EF, Price LH, Kosten TR, Jatlow PI. Cocaethylene: pharmacology, physiology and behavioral effects in humans. *J Pharmacol Exp Ther* 1995;**274**:215–33.

Morton WA. Cocaine and psychiatric symptoms. *Prim Care Companion J Clin Psychiatry* 1999;**1**:109–13.

Pennings EJM, Leccese AP, Wolff FAd. Effects of concurrent use of alcohol and cocaine. *Addiction* 2002;**97**:773–83.

Ruttenber AJ, Lawler-Hernandez J, Yin M, et al. Fatal excited delirium following cocaine use: epidemiologic findings provide new evidence for mechanisms of cocaine toxicity. *J Forensic Sci* 1997;**42**:25–31.

Siegel RK. Cocaine use and driving behavior. *Alcohol Drugs Driv* 1987;**3**:1–7.

White SM, Lambe CJT. The pathophysiology of cocaine abuse. *J Clin Forensic Med* 2003;**10**:27–39.

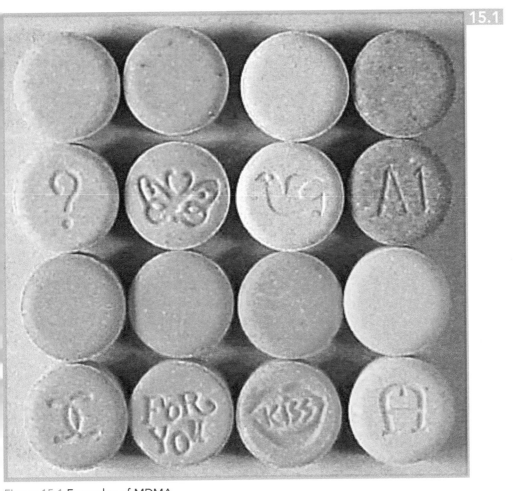

ECSTASY

Principal drugs

3,4–Methylenedioxymethamphetamine (MDMA), 3,4–methylenedioxyethamphetamine (MDEA), 3,4–methylenedioxyamphetamine (MDA) (see also Chapter 9). Some other similar compounds may also be referred to as 'Ecstasy' including PMA and PMMA for which see 'Amphetamine-type Stimulants'.

These drugs (Figure 15.1) are used recreationally, typically in the club and dance culture, for their central stimulant and psychedelic properties resulting in euphoria, and dissociative and empathogenic effects.

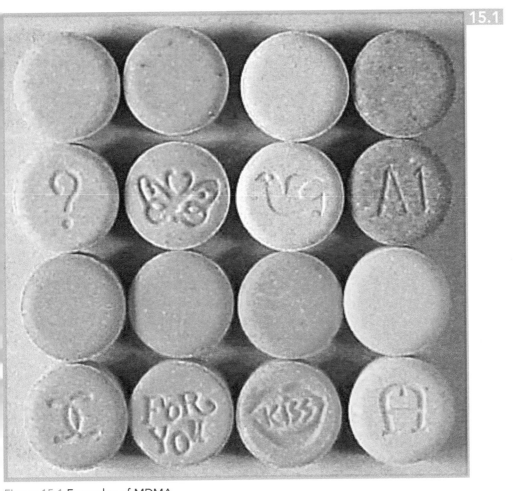

Figure 15.1 **Examples of MDMA.**

Manufacture

Laboratory/factory production.

Common street names

Ecstasy, E, XTC, doves, Dennis, Adam (MDMA), Eve (MDEA).

Mechanism of action

These drugs are powerful central nervous system (CNS) stimulants with mild hallucinogenic properties. MDMA acts predominantly on presynaptic 5-hydroxytryptamine 2 ($5HT_2$) receptors and increases the activity of serotonin, dopamine, and noradrenaline. Compared with the very potent stimulant methamphetamine, MDMA causes greater serotonin release and somewhat lesser dopamine release. Serotonin is a neurotransmitter that plays an important role in the regulation of mood, sleep, pain, emotion, appetite and other behaviours. The excess release of serotonin by MDMA is most probably responsible for the elevation of mood. However, by releasing large amounts of serotonin, MDMA causes the brain to become significantly depleted of this important neurotransmitter, contributing to the negative behavioural after-effects that users often experience for several days after taking MDMA.

Medical uses

Nil. MDMA was previously used in psychotherapeutic settings.

Legal status

Class A under schedule 2 of the Misuse of Drugs Act 1971 (1977 Modification Order).

Presentation and methods of administration

Tablets, which are of variable colours, frequently with a logo (e.g. dove, Mitsubishi, smiley face, star), capsules and, more recently, crystalline powders. Dosages are difficult to quantify owing to the large range of synthetic byproducts and additives often used in preparation (e.g. caffeine, amphetamine analogues, ketamine). Occasionally tablets sold as containing MDMA do not contain any of the drug at all. MDEA is currently rarely encountered. Generally Ecstasy is taken by mouth, and only very rarely injected, snorted or smoked.

Symptoms and signs

Acute intoxication

Physical: effects take up to 1 hour to appear after ingestion and may last for several hours. These are dose dependent – a moderate dose being between 75 and 100 mg; symptoms include tachycardia, dry mouth and throat, jaw clenching and grinding, sweating, pyrexia, nausea and vomiting, transient anorexia, loss of coordination, headache, fatigue, trismus, nystagmus, blurring of vision, ataxia, muscle cramps, urinary urgency, brisk reflexes and paraesthesia.

In overdose or in susceptible individuals, convulsions, hyper- or hypotension, hyperthermia, cardiac dysrhythmias, disseminated intravascular coagulation, rhabdomyolysis and renal failure have been reported. Deaths have been reported in association with the use of single tablets (not caused by contaminants, as has been suggested). Some deaths have been related to cerebral oedema (secondary to excess water ingestion), because the drug has an antidiuretic effect on the kidney. The effects may be exacerbated or precipitated by associated physical activity, e.g. dancing in a hot environment within a club.

Psychological: a mild, euphoric 'rush', feelings of energy and vitality, increased self-esteem, increased self-confidence, feeling of empathy with others, visual and auditory hallucinations (rarely unpleasant); flashbacks may occur, and anxiety attacks, aggression, insomnia or psychosis.

General/chronic

Physical: as for acute intoxication. Physical dependence is not generally considered to occur, although tolerance does occur. Liver abnormalities have been reported. Impairment of cognitive ability has been reported.

Psychological: as for acute intoxication. Flashbacks may be increasingly experienced. Psychological dependence is not believed to occur.

Cessation/withdrawal

After the acute effects of the drug have worn off, the user may experience several days of anxiety, depression and fatigue, variously described as a 'weekend high followed by a midweek low'. Rebound effects include exhaustion, apathy, depression, irritability and insomnia.

Driving

The initial stimulant effects typically last up to 4 h with residual after-effects lasting up to 12 h or more, or often until the person has slept. The stimulant effects, which are very similar to those produced by amphetamine, include increased wakefulness, increased self-confidence and a feeling of physical wellbeing. The reported side or adverse effects include thirst and dilated pupils of the eyes.

The after-effects of the drug are reported to include physical exhaustion, drowsiness, anxiety, agitation and disorientation, which may last for 48 h or more after ingestion of the drug.

The use of stimulant drugs can be associated with risk-taking while the person is experiencing the direct stimulant effects of the drug, e.g. pulling out in front of vehicles where there would normally be insufficient time to do so, or driving faster than normal. It has, however, been reported that acute use of stimulant drugs in low dosage by tired individuals can produce an improvement in attention for a short period of time, with subsequent improvement in performance of certain tasks compared with the situation where no drug has been taken. However, the effect is short-lived.

It is reported that basic vehicle control is only moderately affected. There are, however, indications that under the influence of MDMA individuals accept higher levels of risk. Others have concluded that MDMA use should be considered inconsistent with safe driving immediately following ingestion and for up to a day or longer following use.

Treatment

Intoxication: close observation of pulse rate, blood pressure, temperature and mental state. If any of these are abnormal, observation should be within a hospital setting where facilities for supportive treatment (e.g. ventilation, intracranial pressure monitoring) are readily available. Serotonin syndrome is a possibility, especially if another drug producing serotonin, or preventing reuptake, is ingested. Treatment with benzodiazepines and i/v fluids may be appropriate.

Further reading

Baggott M, Jerome L, Stuart R. 3,4-Methylenedioxymethamphetamine (MDMA): A review of the English-language scientific and medical literature. Original investigator's brochure for MDMA. Multidisciplinary Association for Psychedelic Studies, 2001. Available at: www.maps.org/research/mdma/protocol/mdmareview.pdf (accessed 10 February 2014).

Bosker WM, Kuypers KPC, Conen S, et al. MDMA (ecstasy) effects on actual driving performance before and after sleep deprivation as function of dose and concentration in blood and oral fluid. *Psychopharmacology* 2012;**222**:367–76.

De Waard D, et al. A driving simulator study on the effects of MDMA (Ecstasy) on driving performance and traffic safety. In: Brookhuis KA, Pernot LMC (eds), *Proceedings of the International Council on Alcohol, Drugs and Traffic Safety*. Stockholm: International Council on Alcohol, Drugs and Traffic Safety, 2000.

Jansen KLR. Ecstasy (MDMA) Dependence. *Drug Alcohol Depend* 1999;**53**:121–4.

Logan BK, Couper FJ. 3,4-Methylenedioxymethamphetamine – effects on human performance and behavior. *Forensic Sci Rev* 2003;**15**:12–28.

Morgan MJ. Recreational use of 'ecstasy' (MDMA) is associated with elevated impulsivity. *Neuropsychopharmacology* 1998;**19**:252–64.

Morgan MJ, McFie L, Fleetwood LH, Robinson JA. Ecstasy (MDMA): are the psychological problems associated with its use reversed by prolonged abstinence? *Psychopharmacology* 2002;**159**:294–303.

Morland J. Toxicity of drug abuse – amphetamine designer drugs (ecstasy): mental effects and consequences of single dose use. *Toxicol Lett* 2000;**112–113**:147–52.

Schifano F. Dangerous driving and MDMA ('Ecstasy') abuse. *J Serotonin Res* 1995;**1**:53–7.

Schifano F, Oyefeso A, Corkery J, et al. Death rates from ecstasy (MDMA, MDA) and polydrug use in England and Wales 1996–2002. *Hum Psychopharmacol Clin Exp* 2003;**18**:519–24.

Shulgin AT. The background and chemistry of MDMA. *J Psychoact Drugs* 1986;**8**:291–304.

Steele TD, McCann UD, Ricaurte GA. 3,4-methylenedioxymethamphetamine (MDMA, 'Ecstasy'): pharmacology and toxicology in animals and humans. *Addiction* 1994;**89**:539–51.

γ-HYDROXYBUTYRATE AND RELATED COMPOUNDS

Principal drugs

γ-Hydroxybutyrate (GHB); γ-butyrolactone (GBL); 1,4-butanediol (BD).

Common street names

GHB: Liquid E, Liquid X, Liquid Ecstasy, Easylay, GBH, Grievous bodily harm, Georgia home boy, salt water.

GBL: Blue nitro, Gamma BL, Miracle clean, Midnight blue, Paint stripper, Wax stripper, Video cleaner.

BD: Pine needle oil/extract, Miracle cleaning products, Herbal GHB.

All three drugs are chemically closely related. GHB and GBL can be interconverted by simply changing the acidity or alkalinity of the solution.

The observed effects of all three substances are indistinguishable.

Mechanism of action

They are anaesthetic with a sedative rather than an analgesic effect. GHB is a naturally occurring substance related structurally to GABA (γ-aminobutryic acid) and may be an inhibitory neurotransmitter.

Effects commence between 10 min and an hour after ingestion; if taken in high dosage the effects may last for several hours. Peak plasma levels are achieved within an hour; the drugs have a very short half-life of only 20-60 min or so and, due to their chemical structures, are rarely part of routine drug-testing or drug screening procedures. Specific procedures will be able to detect the drugs only up to a few hours in blood and perhaps up to 8–12 h in urine.

Medical uses

GHB has been used as a premedicant. More recently GHB has been licensed for use in the UK, as the sodium salt, sodium oxybate (Xyrem), to treat narcolepsy with associated cataplexy. GBL and BD have no medical uses.

Legal status

GHB, GBL and BD are all controlled under the Misuse of Drugs Act 1971, class C.

Presentation and methods of administration

Sodium oxybate: oral solution 500 mg/mL.

Illicit: colourless liquids often sold in small bottles. GBL has a chemical/solvent odour. GHB may also be available in powder or capsules, but it rapidly absorbs water to become damp and sticky. The strength of liquids can vary greatly from virtually pure to much less so. GHB is often sold in a clear liquid at around 20% purity. It is taken orally, often as spoon- or capfuls, rarely injected. Although implicated in drug-facilitated sexual assaults the drug has rarely been detected in such cases. The drugs are used widely within the club and dance scene and by body builders because GHB is reported to influence growth hormone levels.

Symptoms and signs

Acute intoxication

Physical effects depend on the dose taken. At low-to-moderate dosage (1–2 g) there is euphoria initially, then sedation, nausea and vomiting, profuse sweating, stiffening of muscles and disorientation; at higher doses (upwards of 2 g) there is ataxia, convulsions, delirium, visual disturbances, coma, bradycardia, hypotension, Cheyne–Stokes respiration and respiratory collapse. The effects can wear off very quickly, although 'hangover' effects may persist for longer. There is a narrow margin between euphoric intoxication and coma, and the effects are worse when mixed with other central nervous system depressants, especially alcohol.

Long-term effects

Unknown, but physical and psychological dependence may occur. Withdrawal effects include anxiety, delirium, confusion, paranoia and possibly psychosis for regular, heavy GHB users, which can last many days – similar to the symptoms and signs of alcohol withdrawal. A rapid deterioration into delirium may occur, especially in more frequent high-dose-dependent users. Withdrawal may be treated with benzodiazepines.

Driving

GHB and GBL can significantly affect driving ability for several hours. Erratic driving may draw attention and drivers have often been found slumped over the steering wheel. Observed effects will be similar to alcohol intoxication and may include dilated pupils, confusion, incoordination, slurred speech and drowsiness, with possible drifting in and out of consciousness after a high dosage. Poor performance on field impairment tests may be expected but the individual may improve rapidly as the drug effects wear off.

Treatment

Diagnosis of intoxication depends on a history of usage together with consistent symptoms over an appropriate time course. There are no specific treatments, although usual basic life support such as maintenance of airway and prevention of vomit aspiration are important.

Further reading

Advisory Council on the Misuse of Drugs. *GBL & 1,4-BD: Assessment of risk to the individual and communities in the UK*. London: ACMD, 2008. Available from: www.homeoffice.gov.uk/acmd1/report-on-gbl1?view=Binary (accessed 20 March 2013).

Andresen H, Aydin BE, Mueller A, Iwersen-Bergmann S. An overview of gamma-hydroxybutyric acid: pharmacodynamics, pharmacokinetics, toxic effects, addiction, analytical methods, and interpretation of result. *Drug Test Anal* 2011;**3**:560–8.

Couper FJ, Marinetti LJ. Gamma-hydroxybutyrate (GHB) – effects on human performance and behavior. *Forensic Sci Rev* 2002;**14**:102–21.

Galloway GP, Frederick-Osborne SL, Seymour R, et al. Abuse and therapeutic potential of gamma-hydroxybutyric acid. *Alcohol* 2000;**20**:263–9.

Jones AW, Holmgren A, Kugelberg FC. Driving under the influence of gamma-hydroxybutyrate (GHB). *Forensic Sci Med Pathol* 2008;**4**:205–11.

Miotto K, Darakjian J, Basch J, et al. Gamma-hydroxybutyric acid: patterns of use, effects and withdrawal. *Am J Addictions* 2001;**10**:232–41.

Scott-Ham M, Burton FC. Toxicological findings in cases of alleged drug-facilitated sexual assault in the United Kingdom over a 3-year period. *J Clin Forensic Med* 2005;**12**:175–86.

Zvosec DL, Smith SW, Porrata T, et al. Case series of 226 γ-hydroxybutyrate-associated deaths: lethal toxicity and trauma. *Am J Emerg Med* 2011;**29**:319–32.

KETAMINE

Principal drugs and derivatives

Ketamine, methoxetamine (N-ethyl derivative of ketamine).

Common street names

Ketamine: special K, vitamin K, K, ket, kit-kat, animal tranquilliser, horse tranquilliser.

Methoxetamine: m-kat, kmax, MXE, mexxy, legal ketamine.

Mechanism of action

Dissociative anaesthetic with analgesic and psychedelic properties, central nervous system (CNS) depressants. Ketamine is a non-competitive N-methyl-D-aspartate (NMDA) receptor antagonist that interferes with the excitatory amino acids including glutamate and aspartate. Oral effects start within 10–20 min and can last up to 3 h; intravenous effects are experienced within 30 seconds and usually last approximately 30 min; insufflation/snorting effects commence within 5–10 min. The half-life of ketamine is 3–4 h.

Medical uses (ketamine)

Intravenous general anaesthetic agent.

There are no medical uses for methoxetamine.

Legal status

Ketamine is a prescription-only medicine, controlled under the Misuse of Drugs Act 1971, class C in 2006, upgraded to class B in June 2014.

Methoxetamine has been controlled as a class B drug since February 2013.

Presentation and methods of administration

Ketamine: sold in liquid form as an anaesthetic, e.g. Ketalar in 10, 50 and 100 mg/mL solutions. Ketamine hydrochloride is found on the 'street' in powder or tablets. It can be taken orally, or by intranasal, intramuscular or intravenous routes.

Methoxetamine: encountered in powder form. Used by nasal insufflation, intravenous and intramuscular injection, sublingually and rectally.

Symptoms and signs

Acute intoxication

Physical: cocaine-like rush, vomiting and nausea, slurred speech, nystagmus, ataxia, loss of coordination, pronounced analgesia, numbness, cardiorespiratory stimulant in low doses, with an increase in blood pressure and pulse. Methoxetamine may have greater potency than ketamine and the effects may last longer.

High doses given by rapid intravenous injection may result in the depression of respiration, or apnoea (which is especially dangerous with other CNS depressants), hypertension, tachycardia and neurological toxicity.

Rarely, depression of the laryngeal reflexes predisposes to aspiration and airway obstruction from inhalation of gastric contents.

Psychological: euphoria, psychological dissociation with hallucinations, anxiety, 'out-of-body' experiences (the 'K-hole').

Chronic

Little information is available, but there may be interference with memory, learning and attention. The user may experience flashbacks. There is no physical dependence or withdrawal. Significant bladder damage is being increasingly reported with signs such as ulcers and fibrosis; pain, urinary incontinence and bleeding can occur. It may be necessary to remove the bladder. This effect has only recently become apparent. There is no evidence yet as to the possible effects on the bladder of methoxetamine.

Driving

Ketamine may impair driving ability for a few hours and can produce distorted perceptions of space and time, decreased awareness of surroundings, an increase in reaction times and blurred vision. White powder around the nose is a common finding for drivers who have recently used ketamine. Methoxetamine would be expected to act similarly although there have been no controlled driving studies for either drug.

Treatment

After non-medical oral or nasal use all that may be required is rest in a quiet, darkened room.

High doses: intensive observation may be required with mechanical support of respiration. Benzodiazepines may assist treatment of associated anxiety.

Further reading

Burch HJ, Clarke EJ, Hubbard AM, et al. Concentrations of drugs determined in blood samples collected from suspected drugged drivers in England and Wales. *J Forensic Legal Med* 2013;**20**: 278–89.

Cheng WC, Ng KM, Chan KK, Mok VKK, Cheung BKL. Roadside detection of impairment under the influence of ketamine – evaluation of ketamine impairment symptoms with reference to its concentration in oral fluid and urine. *Forensic Sci Int* 2007;**170**:51–8.

Corazza O, Schifano F, Simonato P, et al. Phenomenon of new drugs on the internet: the case of ketamine derivative methoxetamine. *Hum Psychopharmacol* 2012;**27**:145–9.

Hansen G, Jensen SB, Chandresh L, et al. The psychotropic effect of ketamine. *J Psychoactive Drugs* 1988;**20**:419–25.

Hofer KE, Grager B, Muller DM, et al. Ketamine-like effects after recreational use of methoxetamine. *Ann Emerg Med* 2012;**60**:97–9.

Jansen KLR. Non-medical use of ketamine. *BMJ* 1993;**306**:601–2.

Mozayani A. Ketamine – effects on human performance and behaviour. *Forensic Sci Rev* 2002;**14**:123–31.

Shields JE, Dargan PI, Wood DM, et al. Methoxetamine-associated reversible cerebellar toxicity: three cases with analytical confirmation. *Clin Toxicol* 2012;**50**:438–40.

Weiner AL, Viera L, McKay CA, Bayer MJ. Ketamine abusers presenting to the emergency department: a case series. *J Emerg Med* 2000;**18**:447–51.

White PF, Way WL, Trevor AJ. Ketamine – its pharmacology and therapeutic uses. *Anesthesiology* 1982;**56**:119–36.

Winstock AR, Mitcheson L, Gillatt DA, Cottrell AM. The prevalence and natural history of urinary symptoms among recreational ketamine users. *BJU Int* 2012;**110**:1762–6.

Wolff K, Winstock AR. Ketamine – from medicine to misuse. *CNS Drugs* 2006;**20**:199–218.

Wood DM, Davies S, Puchnarewicz M, et al. Acute toxicity associated with the recreational use of the ketamine derivative methoxetamine. *Eur J Clin Pharmacol* 2012;**68**:853–6.

KHAT

Principal drugs and derivatives

Khat is an alkaloid (cathinone) derived from the leaves of the khat (qat) shrub – *Catha edulis*. It originates from the Middle East and East Africa. It is structurally similar to amphetamine (see Chapter 9). Many of the new amphetamine-like synthetic drugs are based on the cathinone chemical structure and are known as synthetic cathinones.

Cathinone is broken down to cathine (norephedrine) and norpseudoephedrine. Norephedrine and norpseudoephedrine are the main urinary metabolites, but with some unchanged cathinone also excreted. Use may be detected in urine within 50 min of ingestion – most is excreted by 24 h, but peak plasma levels are 1–2 h after ingestion. The half-life is 3–6 h.

Manufacture

Cultivated.

Common street names

Khat, qat, chat, catha, qaadka.

Mechanism of action

Central nervous system stimulant although much milder than amphetamine.

Medical uses

None.

Legal status

Cathine and cathinone are class C drugs under schedule 2 of the Misuse of Drugs Act 1971. Khat itself also became a Class C controlled drug in the UK in June 2014.

Presentation and methods of administration

Fresh leaves or stalks of the *Catha edulis* plant are chewed (Figure 18.1). Typically 100–200 g of material may be chewed over 3–4 h. It may be drunk as an infusion of leaves (Abyssinian tea).

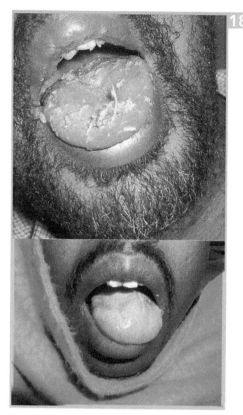

Figure 18.1 Green discoloration and debris on tongue from chewing khat. (JJ Payne-James)

Symptoms and signs

Acute intoxication

Physical: excitable and talkative, anorexia, tachycardia, insomnia, restlessness, dilated pupils reacting slowly to light, hypertension, palpitations, tremor, flushing lasting for up to 3 h. Poor balance. Impotence may be experienced. The mouth and tongue may become inflamed and painful. The tongue may appear green. Gastritis may be present.

Psychological: sense of wellbeing, irritability, euphoria, excitability, agitation, hyperactivity, hypo-/hypermania or lack of concentration, and can stave off hunger.

General/chronic

Long-term use may cause bruxism and a personality change. Psychosis (with visual and auditory hallucinations), although rare, has been reported in predisposed individuals. Paranoid delusions may occur. There may be an increased incidence of peptic ulceration. Khat chewing is a risk factor for increased cerebral haemorrhage, cardiomyopathy and myocardial infarction.

There appears to be little physical dependence but there may be limited psychological dependence, with withdrawal causing some depression and lethargy.

Cessation/withdrawal

Long-term users may experience tremor, lassitude and depression on withdrawal.

Driving

Inattention, impaired judgement and coordination may occur; although khat is reported to produce only limited impairment it may cause drowsiness and apathy later. Green and/or brown-coated tongue and teeth may be present. Drivers have been reported to chew khat to stay awake and improve attention.

Treatment

Intoxication: no specific treatment necessary.

General/chronic: no specific treatment required.

Withdrawal: if withdrawal effects are observed, psychological support and counselling may be required.

Further reading

Chappell JS, Lee MM. Cathinone preservation in khat evidence via drying. *Forensic Sci Int* 2010;**195**:108–20.

Corkery JM, Schifano F, Oyefeso A, et al. Overview of literature and information on 'khat-related' mortality: a call for recognition of the issue and further research. *Ann 1st Super Sanita* 2011;**47**:445–64.

Feigin A, Higgs P, Hellard M, Dietze P. Further research required to determine link between khat consumption and driver impairment. *Bull World Health Organ* 2010;**88**:480.

Giannini AJ, Castellani SJ. A manic-like psychosis due to khat. *J Toxicol Clin Toxicol* 1982;**19**:455–9.

Nencini P, Ahmed AM, Elmi AS. Subjective effects of khat chewing in humans. *Drug Alcohol Depend* 1985;**18**:97–105.

Toennes SW, Kauert GF. Driving under the influence of khat – alkaloid concentrations and observations in forensic cases. *Forensic Sci Int* 2004;**140**:85–90.

LSD

Principal drugs and derivatives

LSD is a semi-synthetic hallucinogen derived from the alkaloid lysergic acid: D-lysergic acid diethylamide, lysergide or LSD-25. Lysergic acid is found in ergot, a fungus which grows on grains such as rye. LSD was first synthesised from lysergic acid in 1938 in Switzerland.

Manufacture

Laboratory/factory production.

Common street names

Acid, tabs, dots, the cube, microdots, pellets, blue star, trips, California sunshine (and also by the names of the designs used in the manufacture of impregnated paper squares e.g. 'Smiley').

Mechanism of action

After oral intake, effects are present within 60 min and last up to 12 h, peaking at about 4 h. It acts on both the central and the autonomic nervous systems. It is metabolised in the liver and kidneys, with faecal excretion. The main site of action is a serotoninergic receptor $5HT_2$. The half-life of lysergide is 3–5 h.

Medical uses

None. When first discovered attempts were made to find a use, particularly in psychiatric disorders.

Legal status

LSD is a class A controlled drug under schedule 1 of the Misuse of Drugs Act 1971.

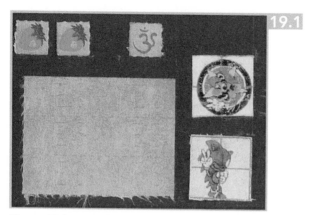

Figure 19.1 **Examples of LSD presentations. (JJ Payne-James)**

Presentation and methods of administration

The amount of LSD required for an effect is very small, typically 25–150 μg being adequate. It may be produced in the form of tablets (microdots), or impregnated on to blotting paper, sugar cubes or gelatine squares (Figure 19.1).

Symptoms and signs

Acute intoxication

Physical: increased blood pressure, pyrexia, headache, dilatation of the pupils, tachycardia. Tremor, flushing, nausea and temporary loss of appetite may be noted. Some temporary muscular incoordination may be experienced.

Psychological: LSD is known as one of the most potent 'mind-expanding' drugs. Both enjoyable and unpleasant effects (a 'bad trip') may be experienced by users. Its effects vary greatly from individual to individual, and may vary in effect in each individual with repeated use. Effects vary with the individual's current state of mind, personality and environment. Visual hallucinations as well as visual distortion may be experienced. Auditory hallucinations are less common. Perception of time may alter, sometimes passing very slowly and sometimes extremely quickly. The ability to judge distance or speed is reduced. Mood may change acutely from extreme happiness to the depths of depression. Paranoia may be felt, and episodes of violence have been described. As the effects of the drug wear off (over a few hours) periods of normality gradually return.

General/chronic

Psychological and physical dependence do not occur because tolerance develops rapidly. There may be an increased risk of spontaneous abortion in pregnant women.

Psychological: prolonged psychotic and anxiety reactions occasionally occur. Flashbacks may occur weeks or months after use.

Cessation/withdrawal

Withdrawal is not considered a problem, because the nature of the drug generally prevents regular daily use.

Driving

Safe control of a motor vehicle is unlikely given the extreme effects that LSD is capable of producing.

Treatment

Intoxication: supportive treatment while 'trip' is under way.

General/chronic: no specific treatment is required. Disturbing flashbacks have been treated with benzodiazepines.

Withdrawal: no specific treatment is required.

Further reading

Hofmann A. The chemistry of LSD and its modifications. In: *LSD A Total Study*. Westbury, NY:PED Publications, 1975.

Passie T, Halpern JH, Stichtinoth DO, et al. The pharmacology of lysergic acid diethylamide: a review. *CNS Neurosci Ther* 2008;**14**:295–314.

Paul BD, Smith ML. LSD – an overview on drug action and detection. *Forensic Sci Rev* 1999;**11**:157–74.

Smart RG, Bateman K. Unfavourable reactions to LSD: a review and analysis of the available case reports. *Can Med Assoc J* 1967;**97**:1214–21.

Smith DE, Seymour RB. Dream becomes nightmare. Adverse reactions to LSD. *J Psych Drugs* 1985;**17**:297–303.

NITRITES

Principal drugs and derivatives

Amyl nitrite, butyl nitrite and isobutyl nitrite.

Manufacture

Laboratory/factory production.

Common street names

Poppers, TNT, nitro, ram, rock hard, rush, liquid gold, locker room.

Mechanism of action

Nitrites dilate blood vessels by relaxing the muscles in the walls of the blood vessels. Inhalation of the vapour results in an almost instantaneous but short-lived effect lasting 15–45 min.

Medical uses

After inhalation nitrites oxidise iron within haemoglobin from the ferrous to the ferric state, forming methaemoglobin. This cannot transport oxygen around the body and, if sufficient nitrite, is ingested it can lead to methaemoglobinaemia. This can be a useful reaction to utilise after cyanide poisoning because cyanide will very effectively bind to methaemoglobin; consequently administration of amyl nitrite, via inhalation, is used as an antidote to cyanide poisoning.

Legal status

Amyl nitrite is classified under the Medicines Act as a pharmacy-only medicine; butyl nitrite is not classified as a drug and therefore there are no restrictions on its availability.

Presentation and methods of administration

Amyl nitrite is a clear, yellow, volatile, inflammable liquid with a sweet pungent smell.

Commercially it is manufactured in a small glass capsule which pops as it is broken open, hence the street name 'poppers'.

As street drugs nitrites are usually encountered in small brown glass bottles, frequently sold as room odourisers. The substance can be inhaled directly from the bottle or poured onto a cloth. Poppers are used to enhance sexual performance and relax the anal sphincter. They are also popular among young people to produce rapid euphoriant effects.

Symptoms and signs

Acute intoxication

Physical: vasodilatation and smooth muscle relaxant, euphoria, cold sweats and hypotension, headache, dizziness, light-headedness, flushed face, weakness, nausea and lacrimation.

Chronic

Signs are facial dermatitis, allergic rash and anaemia. Methaemoglobinaemia may occur. Tolerance does occur but there is no evidence of a physical or psychological dependence.

Driving

The short-lived effects would be incompatible with driving safely when intoxicated.

Treatment

In cases of an overdose remove the person from the exposure and supply oxygen. Serious methaemoglobinaemia may be treated with intravenous methylene blue, e.g. 1.5–2 mg/kg for 5 min together with a litre of intravenous isotonic saline.

Further reading

Lowry TP. Amyl nitrite: an old high comes back to visit. *Behavior Med* 1979;**1**:19–21.

Modarai B, Kapadia YK, Terris J. Methylene blue: a treatment for severe methaemoglobinaemia secondary to misuse of amyl nitrite. *Emerg Med J* 2002;**19**:270–1.

Romanelli F, Smith KM, Thornton AC, Pomeroy C. Poppers: epidemiology and clinical management of inhaled nitrite abuse. *Pharmacotherapy* 2004;**24**:69–78.

Williams JF, Storck M, et al, American Academy of Pediatrics Committee on Substance Abuse. Inhalant abuse. *Pediatrics* 2007;**119**:1009–17.

OPIATES/OPIOIDS

Principal drugs

Opiate drugs are derived from the opium plant and include heroin, morphine, codeine and thebaine. Opioids are analogues to these plant-based drugs but are synthetic, (e.g. methadone and fentanyl) or semi-synthetic (e.g. buprenorphine).

Morphine (MST Continus, Oramorph, Cyclimorph) is a strong analgesic prescribed to treat severe pain and is often used in palliative care.

Codeine and dihydrocodeine(DHC, DF118) are analgesics used to treat mild to moderate pain, with codeine also being used as a cough suppressant and to treat diarrhoea. Both also occur in combination with other drugs e.g. paracetamol in Co-codamol and Co-dydramol.

Oxycodone (Oxycontin, Oxynorm, Percocet) is an analgesic used to treat moderate to severe pain and may also be used in palliative care.

Methadone hydrochloride (Physeptone) is a synthetic opioid analgesic used widely as a treatment of opioid dependence and occasionally for severe pain.

Buprenorphine (Subutex, Temgesic) is an opioid receptor partial agonist/antagonist and is used in the treatment of opiate dependence.

Suboxone is a combination of buprenorphine and naloxone (as 2 mg/0.5mg or 8 mg/2mg), licensed as a substitution treatment for opioid dependence. When administered by dissolution under the tongue, as prescribed, (delete and) very little naloxone reaches the bloodstream because of first-pass metabolism. However, when administered intravenously to opioid-dependent individuals, the naloxone produces marked opioid antagonist effects and causes opioid withdrawal. This acts as a deterrent to intravenous use.

Tramadol (Zamadol, Zydol) is a mixed-action drug with analgesic effects produced by a combination of weak opioid action and a noradrenergic and serotonin mechanism. It is used to treat moderate to severe pain but has also recently been subject to misuse (abuse).

Fentanyl is a strong analgesic normally used as a patch applied to the skin for transdermal drug transfer to treat chronic intractable pain but recommended for use only in opioid tolerant patients.

Dextromoramide (Palfium) was previously used to treat severe pain but is no longer available in the UK.

Dextropropoxyphene (Distalgesic), and when combined with paracetamol (Co-proxamol), were also used to treat moderate to severe pain but are also no longer prescribed to new patients in the UK.

Pentazocine (Fortran) is used rarely to treat moderate to severe pain.

Dipipanone, with cyclizine (Diconal), is used to treat moderate to severe pain although is now only available in the non-proprietary form in the UK.

Recently (2013) a new synthetic opioid, AH-7921, has been encountered as a new psychoactive substance and more might be expected to appear.

Common street names

Heroin: skag, smack, gear, shit

Methadone: amps, linctus, jungle juice

Buprenorphine: subbies, bupe, temmies

Oxycodone: oxy, hillbilly heroin

Dipipanone: dikes

Mechanism of action

Opiates and opioids are analgesics that depress the central nervous system (CNS) through suppression of noradrenaline; when withdrawal occurs there is a rebound release of noradrenaline. They can be categorised by the specific receptor with which the drug interacts and whether the interaction is agonistic, antagonistic or mixed. Pure agonists include morphine and methadone, pure antagonists naltrexone and mixed agonists/antagonists include pentazocine.

Medical uses

Uses of opiates and opioids include for pain relief, as cough suppressants and anti-diarrhoeal agents, and for treatment of opiate dependence (methadone and buprenorphine).

Legal status

They are prescription-only medicines, controlled under the Misuse of Drugs Act 1971. It is illegal to possess them without a prescription. Morphine, opium, methadone, dipipanone, dextromoramide, oxycodone, fentanyl and pethidine are in class A of the Act, dihydrocodeine, codeine and pentazocine in class B, and dextropropoxyphene, tramadol and buprenorphine in class C (see Chapter 3). In June 2014 the UK's ACMD recommended that AH-7921 be included within class A of the Act.

Presentation and methods of administration

Tablets, linctus, injectable liquid if manufactured; illicit powders.

Heroin can be smoked, sniffed or injected (as 'brown', i.e. heroin base powder, heroin will need to be dissolved in an acid, usually citric or ascorbic acid, before intravenous injection; Figure 21.1); most other preparations can be injected or taken orally. Intravenous injection of heroin (mainlining) results in an almost instantaneous effect or 'rush', whereas injection into muscle, or subcutaneously (skin popping), gives a slower and less intense effect. Sniffing will also result in a less intense effect, but the effects of smoking ('chasing the dragon') are almost as quick as an intravenous injection.

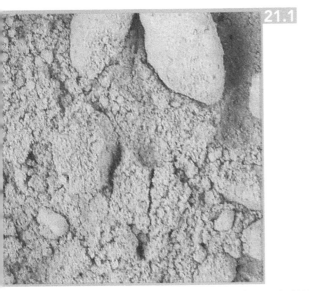

Figure 21.1 **Appearance of powdered heroin ('brown'). (JJ Payne-James)**

Medicinal preparations include the following:

- *Morphine*: tablets and capsules including sustained release 5, 10, 15, 30, 60, 100 and 200 mg; oral solutions, injection ampoules (1 mg/mL, 10 mg/mL), suppositories. Variable onset and duration of effects depending on formulation taken.
- *Methadone*: tablets containing methadone hydrochloride 5 mg; methadone mixture (1 mg/mL), a viscous syrupy liquid, which can be colourless or coloured, containing methadone hydrochloride. A blue hyperconcentrated solution may also be available at 10 mg/mL; a weaker form, methadone linctus, is available at a strength of 2 mg/5 mL; methadone injection clear, colourless liquid in ampoules of 1 mL, 2 mL, 3.5 mL and 5 mL containing methadone hydrochloride BP 10 mg/mL.
- *Oxycodone*: tablets at strengths of 5, 10, 20, 40 or 80 mg; oral solutions 5 mg/5 mL, 10 mg/mL and injection ampoules.
- *Buprenorphine*: tablets 200 μg or 400 mg, injection ampoules 300 mg, and patches 5, 10 or 20 mg/h for 7 days. It is a partial agonist with a long duration of action. It is an effective analgesic and can be taken sublingually or by injection.
- *Fentanyl*: patch 12 or 25 μg per hour (replaced after 72 hours); buccal and sublingual tablets 100, 200, 300, 400, 600, 800 μg
- *Tramadol*: tablets and capsules 50 mg; sustained release 50 or 100mg.

Symptoms and signs

Acute intoxication

Physical: pinpoint (constricted) pupils, depression of the heart rate and respiration, suppression of the cough reflex, constipation, drowsiness and sleep. Nausea and vomiting can occur. High doses can result in respiratory arrest, unconsciousness and death.

Complications may arise due to impurities injected with illicit heroin (including anthrax). Media reports of deaths due to 'contaminated' heroin are normally incorrect and fatality has usually been caused by a batch of heroin with higher than normal purity reaching the end-user. Smoking heroin is a safer mode of use than injection.

Psychological: opioids reduce anxiety, produce pain relief and euphoria, a feeling of contentment and an inability to concentrate. There is little interference with mental or physical functioning. The general depressant effects of opioids may be enhanced by other agents with CNS depressant activity such as alcohol, benzodiazepines, tricyclic antidepressants and phenothiazines. Heroin and/or methadone and alcohol together are a particularly dangerous combination.

Chronic

Tolerance and physical and psychological dependence occur. However, tolerance does not develop to all the effects of opiates because increasing doses have to be taken to achieve the same analgesic or euphoric effect, although pupillary constriction will usually remain constant. Cross-tolerance does occur between the various opiates. If drug administration is stopped, e.g. by a period of imprisonment, tolerance will be lost and there is a risk that, if the previous dose is taken, fatal intoxication can occur. The severity of physical dependence depends on the particular opiate used, the dose and the duration of administration. Psychological dependence on opiates is severe and persists after the physical withdrawal syndrome has passed. There is therefore a high relapse rate of opiate dependence.

Amenorrhoea, loss of libido and chronic constipation occur. Women generally remain fertile despite the menstrual irregularity. Opiate use during pregnancy may result in 'small-for-dates' babies who themselves may suffer severe withdrawal syndrome after birth.

Withdrawal

The onset, peak and duration of symptoms of the withdrawal syndrome will depend on which opiate is misused, e.g. heroin withdrawal will have an earlier onset, and be of shorter duration and greater intensity when compared with methadone. The expectation of withdrawal and psychological factors are also important. Effects start within 8–24 h after the last dose and may last up to 10 days. After chronic administration of buprenorphine the onset of the withdrawal syndrome is delayed, with only mild signs from 3–10 days.

Symptoms: yawning, feelings of hot and cold, anorexia, abdominal cramps, nausea, vomiting, diarrhoea, tremor, insomnia, generalised aches and weakness.

Signs: dilated pupils, gooseflesh, flushing, sweating, rhinorrhoea or lacrimation, tachycardia (a pulse rate of 10 beats/min over the baseline or >90 beats/min if no history of tachycardia), hypertension (systolic blood pressure ≥10 mmHg above baseline or >160/96 in non-hypertensive patients), increased bowel sounds and restlessness.

An opiate withdrawal scale may be useful in certain settings to determine the degree of withdrawal and assess response to therapy (see Appendix D).

Opiate withdrawal during pregnancy can result in fetal death and premature labour. Therefore maintenance therapy with substitute opioids is preferred.

Driving

All opioid drugs are capable of producing effects such as drowsiness, lack of concentration, lack of coordination and slowed reaction times, resulting in poor performance on tasks requiring divided attention, including driving. The effects on any particular individual's driving ability will depend on factors such as how much is taken, the method of administration and the person's tolerance to the drug.

Some of the longer-acting drugs, such as methadone, may not adversely affect driving ability once a person is maintained on a regular daily dose. Codeine, dihydrocodeine, oxycodone and tramadol are only likely to produce significant adverse effects if taken in excessive dosage. Use of heroin is not compatible with safe driving.

Treatment

Overdose: naloxone is a specific opioid antagonist and is given in a dose of 0.4 mg, which can be repeated at intervals of 2–3 min up to a maximum of 10 mg. If there is no effect then the diagnosis of opiate overdose should be reconsidered. Naloxone has a short half-life, so observation in hospital is required after treatment. Naloxone can be given intravenously or intramuscularly (it may be difficult to establish intravenous access) where it is has a longer duration of action.

Naloxone administration is not without risk in the opiate-dependent individual and it may precipitate the opiate withdrawal syndrome, which is distressing but short-lived. Rarely hypertension, pulmonary oedema and cardiac dysrhythmias may occur.

Naltrexone is a specific opioid antagonist in tablet form and is used as an adjunctive therapy in the maintenance of detoxified former opioid-dependent patients.

Withdrawal

The drugs in Table 21.1 can be used in the symptomatic treatment of opiate withdrawal.

Substitution for heroin can be used with a variety of drugs – methadone, buprenorphine, codeine or dihydrocodeine are examples (Table 21.2).

If there is doubt about the daily dose of methadone, this can be divided and the condition of the patient reviewed after a proportion has been administered.

Naltrexone is a pure opiate antagonist with a long half-life. It can be taken orally and blocks the effects of opiates for 72 h, so it can be administered three times a week. It should not be given to an individual who is still dependent on opiates until 7–10 days after the last ingestion of opiates, otherwise it will precipitate a withdrawal reaction that will be protracted because of naltrexone's long duration of action.

Table 21.1 **Symptomatic treatment of opiate withdrawal**

Vomiting	
Prochlorperazine	One or two 3 mg tablets absorbed from buccal cavity twice daily. Useful if unable to retain oral medication
Metoclopramide	One 10 mg tablet three times daily. Not known to be harmful in pregnancy. Action antagonised by opioid analgesics
Abdominal cramps	
Mebeverine	Antispasmodic, not known to be harmful in pregnancy; 135 mg three times daily preferably 20 min before meals
Diarrhoea	
Loperamide	An opiate receptor agonist that acts on the gut to reduce peristalsis, increase intestinal transit time and increase the tone of the anal sphincter. Give two 2 mg capsules initially followed by one after each loose stool; maximum eight daily
Minor aches and pains	
Paracetamol or NSAID*, e.g. ibuprofen	Paracetamol: 1 g up to four times daily. Not known to be harmful in pregnancy
	Ibuprofen: initially 200–400 mg three or four times daily; maximum 2.4 g daily. Avoid NSAIDs in pregnancy, especially in the third trimester
Insomnia	
Zopiclone	Non-benzodiazepine acting at the benzodiazepine receptor, with lower incidence of dependency than benzodiazepines. Short duration of action so less likelihood of 'hangover' effect 7.5 mg at night. *Elderly people*: initially 3.75 mg at night, increased if necessary

*NSAID, non-steroidal anti-inflammatory drug.

From Faculty of Forensic and Legal Medicine and Royal College of Psychiatrists. *Substance Misuse Detainees in Police Custody. Guidelines for Clinical Management*, 4th edn. Report of a Medical Working Group. Council report CR169, London: Royal College of Psychiatrists, 2011. Available from: www.fflm.ac.uk (accessed 5 June 2013).

Table 21.2 Opioid equivalents for withdrawal: related potencies for withdrawal protocols equivalent to 1 mg methadone

Drug:	Dose:
Codeine	15 mg
Dextromoramide	0.5–1 mg
Dextropropoxyphene	15–20 mg
Dihydrocodeine	10 mg
Dipipanone (Diconal)	2 mg
Pharmaceutical heroin	1–2 mg
Hydromorphone	0.5 mg
Methadone linctus	1 mg/2.5 mL
Methadone mixture	1 mg/mL
Morphine	3 mg
Pethidine	15 mg
Buprenorphine[a]	40 μg
Pentazocine[a]	10 mg
Gee's Linctus	10 mL (1.6 mg morphine)
J Collis Brown	10 mL (1 mg extract of opium)

From Faculty of Forensic and Legal Medicine and Royal College of Psychiatrists. *Substance Misuse Detainees in Police Custody. Guidelines for Clinical Management,* 4th edn. Report of a Medical Working Group. Council report CR169, London: Royal College of Psychiatrists, 2011. Available from: www.fflm.ac.uk (accessed 5 June 2013).

Further reading

Bachs LC, Engeland A, Morland JG, Skirtveit S. The risk of motor vehicle accidents involving drivers with prescriptions for codeine or tramadol. *Clin Pharmacol Ther* 2009;**85**:596–9.

Darke S, Duflou J, Torok M. The comparative toxicology and major organ pathology of fatal methadone and heroin toxicity cases. *Drug Alcohol Depend* 2010;**106**:1–6.

Darke S, Zador D. Fatal heroin 'overdose': a review. *Addiction* 1996;**91**:1765–72.

Glare PA, Walsh TD. Clinical pharmacokinetics of morphine. *Ther Drug Monitor* 1991;**13**:1–23.

Gordon NB, Appel PW. Functional potential of the methadone-maintained person. *Alcohol Drugs Driv* 1995;**11**:31–7.

Osborne R, Joel S, Trew D, Slevin M. Morphine and metabolite behavior after different routes of morphine administration: demonstration of the importance of the active metabolite morphine-6-glucuronide. *Clin. Pharmacol Ther* 1990;**47**:12–19.

Pirnay S, Borron SW, Giudicelli CP, Tourneau J, Baud FJ, Ricordel I. A critical review of the causes of death among post-mortem toxicological investigations: analysis of 34 buprenorphine-associated and 35 methadone-associated deaths. *Addiction* 2004;**99**:978–88.

Polettini A, Groppi A, Monagna M. The role of alcohol abuse in the etiology of heroin-related deaths. Evidence for pharmacokinetic interactions between heroin and alcohol. *J Analyt Toxicol* 1999;**23**:570–6.

Schindler S, Ortner R, Peternell A, et al. Maintenance therapy with synthetic opioids and driving aptitude. *Eur Addict Res* 2004;**10**:80–7.

Sporer KA. Acute heroin overdose. *Ann Intern Med* 1999;**130**:584–90.

Stout PR. Farrell LJ. Opioids – effects on human performance and behaviour. *Forensic Sci Rev* 2003; **15**:29–59.

Thiblin I, Eksborg S, Petersson A, Fugelstad A, Rajs J. Fatal intoxication as a consequence of intranasal administration (snorting) or pulmonary inhalation (smoking) of heroin. *Forensic Sci Int* 2004;**139**:241–7.

Vieweg WVR, Lipps WFC, Fernandez A, et al. Opioids and methadone equivalents for clinicians. *J Clin Psychiatry* 2005;**7**:86–8.

Zacny JP. A review of the effects of opiates on psychomotor and cognitive functioning in humans. *Exp Clin Psychopharmacol* 1995;**3**:432–66.

PHENCYCLIDINE

Principal drugs and derivatives

Phencyclidine (PCP)or phencyclidine hydrochloride or 1-[1-phenylcyclohexyl]-piperidine. First developed as an anaesthetic agent in 1959.

Manufacture

Laboratory/factory production; may be diverted from veterinary sources.

Common street names

Angel dust, dust, crystal, rocket fuel. The drug may be mixed with other drugs including crack cocaine (known as 'space base') and cannabis (crystal supergrass, love-boat, killer weed).

Mechanism of action

Dependent on dosage, it may act as an anaesthetic, stimulant, depressant or hallucinogen because it has mixed neurological effects. The drug can cause dissociative effects.

Effects are observed within 30 min if taken orally, but within 5 min if smoked or injected. Acute effects will last for up to 6 h, with a return to normality within 24 h. The half-life is 21 h.

Medical uses

Originally an anaesthetic drug for human and veterinary use. No current medical use.

Legal status

It is a class A drug under schedule 2 to the Misuse of Drugs Act 1971.

Presentation and methods of administration

PCP is a crystalline white powder, readily soluble in water or alcohol. It may be encountered as a liquid, and can be smoked, taken orally or intranasally, or injected intravenously.

Symptoms and signs

Acute intoxication

Physical: at lower to moderate doses (<10 mg) there may be loss of coordination, slurred speech, skin flushing, increased muscle tone, numbness of the limbs and sweating, tachycardia, tachypnoea and hypertension. The user may show a fixed blank stare and repetitive incoherent speech. At higher doses (>10 mg) blood pressure, pulse and respiratory rate may all decrease. Vertical nystagmus, visual disturbance, excessive salivation and nausea may be experienced. The anaesthetic properties of PCP may render the individual less sensitive to pain, allowing injuries to go unnoticed. Death due to convulsions, respiratory arrest and hypertension has been reported.

Psychological: lower doses may cause irritability, euphoria or anxiety and, as doses increase, disturbances of body image, aggression and paranoia can be experienced. Auditory hallucinations will be observed with higher doses and episodes of bizarre behaviour are common. Paranoid delusions become increased and the individual may react to perceived threats with frightening physical violence.

General/chronic

Physical: no physical dependence occurs.

Psychological: there is some evidence that psychological dependence develops. Memory may be affected. Drug-induced psychosis after use of PCP may last up to several weeks, particularly in those with a history of psychiatric disorders such as schizophrenia. Tolerance may develop and craving for the drug may occur.

Cessation/withdrawal

Depression and social withdrawal are common sequelae of chronic PCP misuse. There may be a mild abstinence syndrome with depression and disorientation.

Driving

PCP has been shown to produce significant disorientation, drowsiness, lack of attention and coordination, slowed reaction time and impaired perception of space. These effects may last in excess of 12 h after use.

Treatment

Intoxication: acidification of the urine may reduce the drug half-life by accelerating excretion. Haloperidol has been used and evaluated, orally, intramuscularly and intravenously.

General/chronic: no specific treatment.

Withdrawal: standard treatment(s) for depressive episodes when clinically indicated.

Further reading

Clardy DO, Gravey RH, MacDonald BJ, Wiersma SJ, Pearce, DS, Ragle JL. The phencyclidine-intoxicated driver. *J Analyt Toxicol* 1979;**3**:238–41.

Clouet DH, ed. NIDA Research Monograph 64: Phencyclidine – an update. Department of Health and Human Services, Public Health Service, Alcohol, Drug Abuse, and Mental Health Administration, 1986. Available from: http://archives.drugabuse.gov/pdf/monographs/64.pdf (accessed 3 June 2013).

Kunsman GW, Levine B, Costantino A, Smith ML. Phencyclidine blood concentrations in DRE cases. *J Analyt Toxicol* 1997;**21**:498–502.

McCarron MM, Schulze BW, Thompson GA, Conder MC, Goetz WA. Acute phencyclidine intoxication: incidence of clinical findings in 1,000 cases. *Ann Emerg Med* 1981;**10**:237–42.

McCarron MM, Schulze BW, Thompson GA, Conder MC, Goetz WA. Acute phencyclidine intoxication: clinical patterns, complications and treatment. *Ann Emerg Med* 1981;**10**:290–7.

MacNeal JJ, Cone DC, Sinha V, et al. Use of haloperidol in PCP-intoxicated individuals. *Clin Toxicol* 2012;**50**:851–3.

PHENETHYLAMINES

Principal drugs and derivatives

A wide range of compounds falls within this very broad category of drugs. Within the category the so-called '2C' group comprises phenethylamines with methoxy groups on the 2 and 5 positions of the benzene ring, including:

- 2-CB (4-bromo-2,5-dimethoxyphenethylamine)
- 2-CE (2,5-dimethoxy-4-ethylphenethylamine)
- 2-CI (2,5-dimethoxy-4-iodophenethylamine)
- 25B-NBOMe (4-bromo-2,5-dimethoxy-N-(2-methoxyphenyl)phenethylamine)
- 25I-NBOMe (4-iodo-2,5-dimethoxy-N-(2-methoxyphenyl)phenethylamine)
- 25C-NBOMe (4-chloro-2,5-dimethoxy-N-(2-methoxyphenyl)phenethylamine)
- DOI (2,5-dimethoxy-4-iodo-amphetamine)
- DOM (2,5-dimethoxy-4-methylamphetamine).

Other structurally related drugs include 2CB-FLY (2-(8-bromo-2,3,6,7-tetrahydrofuro [2,3-f][1]benzofuran-4-yl)ethanamine), Bromodragonfly (1-(4-bromofuro[2,3-f] benzofuran-8-yl)propan-2-amine) and mescaline (3,4,5-trimethoxyphenethylamine).

Manufacture

Illicit laboratories; mescaline occurs naturally in the peyote cactus (*Lophophora williamsii*), native to southern North America and the San Pedro cactus (*Echinopsis pachanoi*), native to South America, and a few other plant species.

Common street names

Nexus, bromo, N-bomb, Europa, CBs, bomb-25, smiley paper.

Mechanism of action

These are central nervous system stimulants but often with powerful hallucinogenic effects. They are absorbed by the gastrointestinal tract and may have an effect within 20 min of ingestion. Some compounds have delayed action and some have a very steep dose–response curve, so there can be large differences in effects and duration even with a small variation in dosage.

Active dosages for many of these drugs are very low with as little as 0.1 mg being required for the 'N-bomb' drugs. Others may require up to 5 mg although a typical dose of 2C-B is 10-25 mg. Large dosages of some drugs may produce effects lasting more than 24 h. Half-lives for most of these drugs have not been established.

Medical uses

None

Legal status

Now that the NBOMe series of drugs have recently been controlled (June 2014) all are now class A drugs in the UK.

Presentation and methods of administration

Powders, capsules, tablets, paper squares. Taken orally or by snorting but can be taken sublingually or via injection.

Symptoms and signs

Acute intoxication

Physical: very varied; can include poor coordination, giggling/smiling, muscle spasms, tremors, headache, bruxism, tachycardia, tachypnoea.

Psychological: psychedelic effects, sometimes in waves.

Higher doses can result in irrational behaviour, confusion, fear, hallucinations, delusions, paranoia and psychosis.

General/chronic

Unknown.

Driving

All likely to be incompatible with driving a motor vehicle but no known studies.

Treatment

Intoxication: nil – unless complications develop. Then supportive with monitoring of vital signs in hospital setting; intravenous benzodiazepines may be appropriate.

Further reading

Acuna-Castillo A, Villalobos C, Moya PR, et al. Differences in potency and efficacy of a series of phenylisopropylamine/phenylethylamine pairs at 5-HT(2A) and 5-HT(2C) receptors. *Br J Pharmacol* 2002;**136**:510–19.

de Boer D, Gijzels MJ, Bosman IJ, Maes RA. More data about the new psychoactive drug 2C-B. *J Analyt Toxicol* 1999;**23**:227–8.

McGrane O, Simmons J, Jacobsen E, Skinner C. Alarming trends in a novel class of designer drugs. *J Clin Toxicol* 2011;**1**(2).

Sacks J, Ray MJ, Williams S, et al. Fatal toxic leukoencephalopathy secondary to overdose of a new psychoactive designer drug 2C-E ('Europa'). *Proc (Bayl Med Cent)* 2012;**25**:374–6.

Shulgin AT, Shulgin A. *PiHKAL – A Chemical Love Story.* Berkeley, CA: Transform Press, 1991.

Villalbos CA, Bull P, Saez P, et al. 4-Bromo-2,5-dimethoxyphenethylamine (2C-B) and structurally related phenylethylamines are potent 5-HT2A receptor antagonists in *Xenopus laevis* oocytes. *Br J Pharmacol* 2004;**141**:1167–74.

Wood DM, Looker JJ, Shaikh L, et al. Delayed onset of seizures and toxicity associated with recreational use of bromo-dragonfly. *J Med Toxicol* 2009;**5**:226–9.

Zuba D, Sekula K, Buczek A. 25C-NBOMe – new potent hallucinogenic substance identified on the drug market. Forensic Sci Int 2013;**227**:7–14

PIPERAZINES

Principal drugs and derivatives

1-Benzylpiperazine (BZP), 1-(3-trifluoromethylphenyl)piperazine (TFMPP), 1-(3-chlorophenyl)piperazine (mCPP).

Manufacture

Illicit laboratories; mCPP is a metabolite of trazodone.

Common street names

Legal E, legal X, herbal ecstasy, BZPs, party pills.

Mechanism of action

They are central nervous system stimulants although they are less potent than amphetamine and MDMA. TFMPP produces fewer stimulant effects than BZP and is associated with increased anxiety; mCPP can produce unpleasant effects and is less desirable to users. TFMPP and mCPP may produce hallucinogenic effects.

They are absorbed by the gastrointestinal tract and the effects commence within 20 min of ingestion and last for up to 8 h.

Dosage range is normally up to 200 mg for BZP, but ≤100 mg for TFMPP. BZP and TFMPP are sometimes encountered together e.g. as a 10:1 mix. The half-life for BZP is reported as 5.5 h.

Medical uses

None.

Legal status

They are controlled by the Misuse of Drugs Act 1971, class C in the UK.

Presentation and methods of administration

Powders, capsules, tablets. Taken orally or by snorting; may be injected occasionally.

Symptoms and signs

Acute intoxication

Physical: anxiety, vomiting, sweating, headache and palpitations.

Psychological: difficulties sleeping, mood swings, loss of energy, irritability, confusion. Higher doses can result in unpredictable and serious toxicity including seizures and collapse.

General/chronic

Unknown.

Driving

A study showed that BZP/TFMPP improved driving performance by improving attention and decreasing weaving of the vehicle. However, the study was stopped early due to the high incidence of severe adverse events. including agitation, anxiety, hallucinations, vomiting, insomnia and migraine.

Treatment

Intoxication: nil – unless complications develop. Then treatment is supportive with monitoring of vital signs in a hospital setting; intravenous benzodiazepines may be appropriate.

Further reading

Antia U, Lee HS, Kydd RR, Tingle MD, Russell BR. Pharmacokinetics of 'party pill' drug N-benzylpiperazine (BZP) in healthy human participants. *Forensic Sci Int* 2009;**186**:63–7.

Elliott S. Current awareness of piperazines: pharmacology and toxicology. *Drug Test Anal* 2011;**3**:430–8.

Elliott S, Smith C. Investigation of the first deaths in the United Kingdom involving detection and quantitation of the piperazines BZP and 3-TFMPP. *J Analyt Toxicol* 2008;**32**:172–7.

Gee P, Gilbert M, Richardson S, Moore G, Paterson S, Graham P. Toxicity from the recreational use of 1-benzylpiperazine. *Clin Toxicol* 2008;**46**:802–7.

Lin JC, Jan RK, Kydd RR, Russell BR. Subjective effects in human following administration of party pill drugs BZP and TFMPP alone and in combination. *Drug Test Anal* 2011;**3**:582–5.

Schep LJ, Slaughter RJ, Vale A, Beasley M, Gee GP. The clinical toxicology of the designer 'party pills' benzylpiperazine and trifluoromethylphenylpiperazine. *Clin Toxicol* 2011;**49**:131–41.

Sheridan J, Butler R, Wilkins C, Russell B. Legal piperazines-containing party pills – a new trend in substance misuse. *Drug Alcohol Rev* 2007;**26**:335–43.

Tancer ME, Johanson CE. The subjective effects of MDMA and mCPP in moderate MDMA users. *Drug Alcohol Depend* 2001;**65**:97–101.

Thompson I, William G, Caldwell B, et al. Randomised double-blind, placebo-controlled trial of the effects of the 'party pills' BZP/TFMPP alone and in combination with alcohol. *J Psychopharmacol* 2010;**24**:1299–308.

PIPRADROLS

Principal drugs and derivatives

Desoxypipradrol, diphenylprolinol, diphenylmethylpyrrolidine.

Common street names

D2PM, 2-DPMP, 'Ivory wave', 'Head candy'. Frequently marketed as being 'not for human consumption' and 'research chemicals' in attempts to circumvent the legislation under the Medicines Act 1968.

Mechanism of action

Central nervous system stimulants increasing dopamine release and also decreasing dopamine reuptake. Absorbed by the gastrointestinal tract and effects commence within 20 minutes of oral ingestion with a faster onset if snorted. The effects are long lasting, perhaps several days.

Medical uses

No medical uses at present.

Legal status

The named pipradrols are controlled by the Misuse of Drugs Act 1971 Class B.

Presentation and methods of administration

Tablets, capsules or powder. May be taken orally or snorted. Typical dosage is within a range of 10 to 25mg.

Symptoms and signs

Acute intoxication

Physical: tachycardia, hypertension, sweating, bruxism, agitation, rhabdomyolysis. These effects may last several days but generally wear off of their own accord. Neuropsychiatric effects may last up to a week after ingestion. Deaths have been reported.

Psychological: euphoria, paranoia, psychosis.

General/chronic

Physical: long-term use. No information available.

Psychological: in addition to the short-term effects continued usage could cause aggression, fatigue, weakness, insomnia, anxiety, depression, psychosis.

Cessation/withdrawal

Cessation can cause anxiety and depression, disturbance of sleep patterns, irritability.

Driving

No published controlled studies but would be expected to produce similar effects to other stimulant drugs for example, increased risk-taking, impatience and driving at high speed. Physical signs may include restlessness, agitation and aggression. One paper has published findings in drivers.

Treatment

Intoxication: nil – unless complications develop. Then supportive with monitoring of vital signs in hospital setting. Benzodiazepines may be useful to treat agitation.

General/chronic: as for intoxication.

Withdrawal: psychological support and counselling.

Further reading

Iversen L, White M, Treble R. Designer psychostimulants: pharmacology and differences. *Neuropharmacology* 2014. http://dx.doi.org/10.1016/j.neuropharm. 2014.01.15.

Kriikku P, Wilhelm L, Rintatalo J et al. Prevalence and blood concentrations of desoxypipradrol (2-DPMP) in drivers suspected of driving under the influence of drugs and in post-mortem cases. *Forensic Sci Int* 2013;**226**:146-151.

Lidder S, Dargan P, Sexton M et al. Cardiovascular toxicity associated with recreational use of diphenylprolinol (diphenyl-2-pyrrolidinemethanol [D2PM]). *J Med Toxicol* 2008;**4**:167-169.

Simmler LD, Rickli A, Schramm Y et al. Pharmacological profiles of aminoindanes, piperazines and pipradrol derivatives. *Biochem Pharmacol* 2014;**88**:237-244.

Wood DM, Dargan PI. Use and acute toxicity associated with the novel psychoactive substances diphenylprolinol (D2PM) and desoxypipradrol (2-DPMP). *Clin Toxicol* 2012;**50**:727-732.

SYNTHETIC CANNABINOIDS

Principal drugs and derivatives

WH-018, JWH-022, JWH-073, JWH-122, JWH-210, HU-210, CP47, AM-694, AM-2201, UR-144, PB-22, RCS-4, URB-597, APINACA and very many others. Several hundred different 'spice' compounds have been identified.

Common street names

Spice, spice gold, spice silver, K2, herbal incense, herbal smoking blends, black mamba, annihilation, bliss, fake weed, blaze.

Mechanism of action

Most of these compounds target the CB1 cannabinoid receptor, producing peripheral and central nervous system effects. There is increasing evidence for parent drugs, and metabolites, binding to CB2 cannabinoid receptors. Many are more potent than tetrahydrocannabinol (THC) with JWH-018 having 4x, JWH-122 60x and JWH-210 90x the potency of THC. They are abused for their euphoric, energising and disinhibitory effects. There are few studies of the half-life, but it is probably very short, e.g. JWH-018 about 2 h.

Medical uses

No medical uses.

Legal status

Changes quickly. Currently all listed drugs are controlled by the Misuse of Drugs Act 1971, class B via generic definitions.

Presentation and methods of administration

Normally presented as herbal mixtures with the active ingredient sprayed onto the herbal material, but they are also available as pure compounds.

A typical dosage is <10 mg of active constituent, often 1–2 mg.

Symptoms and signs

Acute intoxication

Physical: tachycardia, hypertension, hallucinations, nausea and vomiting, chest pain, seizures, somnolence, dilated pupils and respiratory depression. Use of spice compounds may lead to presentation at hospitals due to unpleasant and/or frightening effects.

Psychological: acute anxiety, psychosis and memory changes.

General/chronic

As most of these drugs are relatively new on the drug misuse scene, there is little information about longer-term use, although increased risk of psychosis has been reported in users who had smoked the drug between four times over a 3-week period and daily for 18 months. Cognitive impairment has also been reported.

Physical: none described.

Psychological: few data to date but reports of psychoses including episodes of visual and auditory hallucinations, paranoid delusions, anxiety, insomnia and suicidal ideation have been appearing in the literature.

Cessation/withdrawal

Drug craving, nocturnal nightmares, sweating, headache, tremor, nausea.

Driving

There are few studies to date but similar effects to cannabis, including sedation and impairment of fine motor skills, have been reported. Analytical findings in driving cases have also been reported.

Treatment

Intoxication: nil – unless complications develop. Then treatment is supportive with monitoring of vital signs in hospital setting.

General/chronic: as for intoxication.

Withdrawal: psychological support and counselling.

Further reading

Atwood BK, Lee D, Straiker A, et al. CP47, 497-C8 and JWH-073, commonly found in 'Spice' herbal blends, are potent and efficacious CB1 cannabinoid receptor agonists. *Eur J Pharmacol* 2011;**659**:139–45.

Fattore L, Fratta W. Beyond THC: the new generation of cannabinoid designer drugs. *Frontiers Behav Neurosci* 2011;**5**(Article 60):1–12.

Gunderson EW, Haughey HM, Ait-Daoud N, et al. 'Spice' and 'K2' herbal highs: a case series and systematic review of the clinical effects and biopsychosocial implications of synthetic cannabinoid use in humans. *Am J Addict* 2012;**21**:320–6.

Harris CR, Brown A. Synthetic cannabinoid intoxication: A case series and review. *J Emerg Med* 2013;**44**:360–6.

Hermanns-Clausen M, Kneisel S, Szabo B, et al. Acute toxicity due to the confirmed consumption of synthetic cannabinoids: clinical and laboratory findings. *Addiction* 2013;**108**:534–44.

Hudson S, Ramsey J. The emergence and analysis of synthetic cannabinoids. *Drug Test Anal* 2011;**3**:466–78.

Mushoff F, Madea B, Kernbach-Wighton G, et al. Driving under the influence of synthetic cannabinoids ('Spice'): a case series. *Int J Legal Med* 2014;**128**:59–64.

Rajasekaran M, Brents LK, Franks LN, et al. Human metabolites of synthetic cannabinoids JWH-018 and JWH-073 bind with high affinity and act as potent agonists at cannabinoid type-2 receptors. *Toxicol Appl Pharmacol* 2013;**269**:100–8.

Seely KA, Lapoint J, Moran JH, et al. Spice drugs are more than harmless herbal blends; A review of the pharmacology and toxicology of synthetic cannabinoids. *Prog Neuro-Psychopharmacol Biol Psychiatry* 2012;**39**:234–43.

Teske J, Weller JP, Fieguth A, Rothamel T, Schulz Y, Troger HD. Sensitive and rapid quantification of the cannabinoid receptor agonist naphthalen-1-yl-(1-pentylindol-3-yl)methanone (JWH-018) in human serum by liquid chromatography-tandem mass spectrometry. *J Chromatogr B Analyt Technol Biomed Life Sci* 2010;**878**:2659–63.

SYNTHETIC CATHINONES

Principal drugs and derivatives

Mephedrone (4-methylmethcathinone), 4-methylethcathinone, methedrone (4-methoxymethcathinone), MDPV (3,4-methylenedioxy-pyrovalerone), methylone (3,4-methylenedioxy-methylcathinone), butylone (methylenedioxy-phenyl-2-methylaminobutanone), flephedrone (4-fluoromethcathinone), naphyrone (naphthylpyrovalerone) and many others.

Manufacture

Laboratory/factory production.

Common street names

Bath salts, legal highs, plant food, NRG-1, NRG-2, MCAT, ivory wave, miaow-miaow, 4-MMC, 4-MEC, MMCAT, 4-FMC, bubbles, rush. Frequently marketed as being 'not for human consumption' and 'research chemicals' in attempts to circumvent the legislation under the Medicines Act 1968.

It is important to understand that often sellers, buyers and users do not know which of these drugs they are providing or using.

Mechanism of action

These drugs are central nervous system stimulants of varying potency; they also have a psychostimulant action with some effects resembling MDMA. They are absorbed by the gastrointestinal tract and effects commence within 20 min of oral ingestion, faster if snorted. The effect is immediate if injected. The effects last 1–4 h, and the compounds are mostly metabolised by the liver. They are heavily metabolised but some drug may be eliminated unchanged in the urine. Half-lives have not been established.

Medical uses

No medical uses at present.

Legal status

This changes quickly. Currently all listed drugs are controlled by the Misuse of Drugs Act 1971, class B. Recent UK legislation permits quick temporary control (up to a year) if a new and potentially dangerous drug is encountered.

Presentation and methods of administration

Tablets, capsules, powder. May be taken orally, sniffed, snorted, smoked or injected. Typical dosages depend on the specific drug, the route of administration and drug purity e.g. mephedrone dosage may be up to 250 mg if taken orally but 150 mg if snorted; MDPV dosage is much lower being 5 to 20 mg.

Symptoms and signs

Acute intoxication

Physical: low-to-moderate doses may produce tachypnoea, tachycardia, hypertension, loss of appetite, dilatation of pupils, brisk reflexes, fine tremor of limbs, agitation, insomnia, nausea, headache, body odour and memory loss. Higher doses will produce dry mouth, pyrexia, sweating, blurring of vision, dizziness, bruxism, flushing or pallor, cardiac dysrhythmias, loss of coordination, hallucinations, delirium, seizures, paranoia or vomiting. These effects may last several hours depending on the drug used and dosage, but generally wear off of their own accord. Deaths have been reported.

Psychological: euphoria, feeling of self-confidence, raised self-esteem, lowered anxiety, increased energy, greater concentration, empathy, openness, increased libido, irritability, restlessness. Higher doses can result in irrational behaviour, confusion, fear, hallucinations memory loss, delusions, paranoia or psychosis. Psychological dependence has been observed although, as yet, physical dependence is not generally considered to occur. A strong craving to repeat or increase dosage is common.

If injected the user additionally experiences a sensory 'rush' or 'flash' – giving almost immediate sensations of enhanced energy and self-confidence, and enhanced sexual enjoyment.

As these drugs are powerful stimulants with significant effects on neurotransmitters they can lead to development of excited delirium and serotonin syndrome.

General/chronic

Longer-term use may require increased dosage levels due to tolerance. Some of these drugs may be used over a period of days until the supply has been exhausted (provoking comparison with cocaine binges), after which the user may be completely exhausted and consequently sleep for several days.

Physical: long-term use. Little information is currently available because of their only recent increased usage.

Psychological: in addition to the short-term effects, continued usage can cause aggression, fatigue, weakness, insomnia, anxiety, depression, psychosis or increased strength – users may need to be physically restrained.

Cessation/withdrawal

Users find that cessation can cause anxiety and depression, disturbance of sleep patterns and irritability.

Driving

No published controlled driving studies are available. Some studies have published findings in drivers who have taken synthetic cathinones. Synthetic cathinones would be expected to produce similar effects to other stimulant drugs, e.g. increased risk taking, impatience and driving at high speed. Physical signs may include dilated pupils, restlessness, agitation and aggression. The stimulant effects may last 1–4 h. In the comedown phase, lack of attention, poor coordination, drowsiness and slow response times might be expected and may last many hours. These drugs are often taken together with other drugs which will complicate the signs demonstrated.

Treatment

Intoxication: nil – unless complications develop, then supportive with monitoring of vital signs in hospital setting. Benzodiazepines may be useful to treat agitation. Diagnosis and treatment can be complicated by co-ingestion of other drugs (frequency >80%).

General/chronic: as for intoxication.

Withdrawal: psychological support and counselling.

Further reading

Baumann MH, Partilla JS, Lehner KR. Psychoactive "bath salts": not so soothing. *Eur J Pharmacol* 2013;**698**:1–5

Burch HJ, Clarke EJ, Hubbard AM, et al. Concentrations of drugs determined in blood samples collected from suspected drugged drivers in England and Wales. *J Forensic Legal Med* 2013;**20**: 278–89.

Corkery J, Schifano F, Ghodse AH, et al. Mephedrone-related fatalities in the United Kingdom. In: Gallelli L (ed.), *Contextual, Clinical and Practical Issues. Pharmacology.* InTech, 2012.

Cosbey SH, Peters KL, Quinn A, et al. Mephedrone (Methylmethcathinone) in toxicology casework: A Northern Ireland perspective. *J Analyt Toxicol* 2013;**37**:74–82.

Dargan PI, Sedefov R, Gallegos A, et al. The pharmacology and toxicology of the synthetic cathinone mephedrone (4-methylmethcathinone). *Drug Test Anal* 2011;**3**:454–63.

De Felice LJ, Glennon RA, Negus SS. Synthetic cathinones: chemical phylogeny, physiology and neuropharmacology. *Life Sci* 2014;**97**:20–26.

EMCDDA Risk Assessments. *Report on the risk-assessments of mephedrone in the framework of the council decision on new psychoactive drugs.* No. 9. EMCDDA, Lisbon, 2011.

Kelly JP. Cathinone derivatives: a review of their chemistry, pharmacology and toxicology. *Drug Test Anal* 2011;**3**:439–53.

Maskell PD, De Paoli G, Seneviratne C, et al. Mephedrone (4-methylmethcathinone)-related deaths. *J Analyt Toxicol* 2011;**35**:189–91.

Miotto K, Striebel J, Cho AK et al. Clinical and pharmacological aspects of bath salt use: a review of the literature and case reports. *Drug & Alc Depend* 2013;**132**:1–12

Prosser JM, Nelson LS. The toxicology of bath salts: a review of synthetic cathinones. *J Med Toxicol* 2012;**8**:33–42.

Simmler LD, Rickli A, Hoener MC et al. Monoamine transporter and receptor interaction profiles of a new series of designer cathinones. *Neuropharmacol.* 2014;**79**:152–160.

Warrick BJ, Wilson J, Hedge M, Freeman S, Leonard K, Aaron C. Lethal serotonin syndrome after methylone and butylone ingestion. *J Med Toxicol* 2012;**8**:65–8.

TOBACCO

Tobacco is produced from the tobacco plant – *Nicotiana tabacum*.

Principal drugs and derivatives

The content of tobacco smoke is complex. About 500 different compounds have been identified. The main pharmacologically active ingredients are nicotine and tars. Nicotine is an oily alkaloid. Pure nicotine is extremely poisonous – a dose of 50 mg can cause death within minutes.

Manufacture

Tobacco plants are commercially cultivated and harvested worldwide.

Common street names

Ciggies, tabs, roll-ups, fags, smokes, gaspers.

Mechanism of action

Nicotine is both a stimulant and a sedative, with effects on the central nervous and voluntary and involuntary nervous systems that are dose dependent. In the doses used in smoking, nicotine causes release of catecholamines, serotonin, antidiuretic hormone, corticotrophin and growth hormone. Nicotine inhaled as smoke will reach the brain within 1 min. Its effects on the body last for about 30 min. It is excreted in urine after metabolism to inert substances. Cotinine, another component of tobacco but also a metabolite of nicotine, is sometimes used as a marker for tobacco use.

Medical uses

None.

Legal status

Tobacco products may not be sold to those under 18 years of age in the UK.

Presentation and methods of administration

Dried leaves of the tobacco plant may be smoked in cigarettes (manufactured or 'roll-ups'), cigars and pipes. The leaves may be chewed. Ground-up dried tobacco may be taken as snuff. One cigarette may contain up to 20 mg nicotine but lower nicotine brands may be as low as 0.5 mg and ultra-low as low as 0.1 mg. Actual nicotine content may bear little relationship to the amount of nicotine ingested. A cigarette may contain up to 15 mg tar, low-tar brands containing considerably less.

Symptoms and signs

Acute intoxication

Physical: tachycardia, hypertension, sore throat, sore eyes and tremor.

Psychological: some individuals feel more alert and some feel more tranquil.

General/chronic

Physical: physical dependence develops rapidly (within days). Long-term smoking is associated with a large range of diseases and illnesses including lung cancer, atherosclerosis (manifest as angina, myocardial infarction, cerebrovascular accidents or peripheral vascular disease), bronchitis, peptic ulcers, reduced fertility (females), complications of pregnancy (including smaller babies), and cancers of the mouth and throat. Children of female smokers may be shorter and have delayed intellectual development. All these risks increase the longer the individual has smoked. The risks vary according to the type of use (e.g. cigarettes versus pipes) and the method of use (e.g. inhaling versus not inhaling). Stopping smoking will eventually decrease the risk.

Psychological: psychological dependence is marked.

Cessation/withdrawal

A withdrawal syndrome develops with the individual initially experiencing fatigue, shortness of breath and headache, and longer-term agitation, irritability and depression. Many individuals become preoccupied with the absence of smoking. Weight gain may be observed because of a reduction in metabolic rate and 'comfort' eating.

Treatment

Intoxication: no specific treatment.

General/chronic: the ease (or not) of cessation of smoking varies with each individual. Some individuals may stop without support, but most require help. Tapered nicotine replacement therapy (NRT), using nicotine-supplying gum, lozenges, sublingual tablets, skin patches or fake cigarettes, may be useful.

Bupropion (Zyban), an antidepressant, may be used as a treatment over a period of 7–9 weeks, although the mechanism of action is unclear. Varenicline (Champix) is a selective nicotine receptor partial agonist that may also be used in a 12-week cycle of treatment. Anxiolytic drugs, counselling, hypnotherapy and acupuncture all have their place in the management of those experiencing difficulties.

Withdrawal: no specific treatment, except NRT.

Further reading

Moylan S, Jacka FN, Pasco JA, Berk M. Cigarette smoking, nicotine dependence and anxiety disorders: a systematic review of population-based, epidemiological studies. *BMC Med* 2012;**10**:123.

Ueda K, Kawachi I, Nakamura M, et al. Cigarette nicotine yields and nicotine intake among Japanese male workers. *Tobacco Control* 2002;**11**:55–60.

TRYPTAMINES

Principal drugs and derivatives

A wide range of compounds fall within this very broad category of drugs, which includes endogenous compounds such as serotonin (5-hydroxytryptamine) and melatonin, naturally occurring compounds such as psilocybin, bufotenine (5-hydroxydimethyltryptamine), mitragynine, DMT (dimethyltryptamine) and 5-MeO-DMT (5-methoxydimethyltryptamine), and synthetic drugs including AMT (α-methyltryptamine), 5-MeO-DALT (N,N-diallyl-5-methoxytryptamine) and 5-methoxy-N, N-diisopropyltryptamine.

Manufacture

Psilocybin occurs naturally in more than 200 species of mushrooms belonging to the genus *Psilocybe*. One of the most common species is *P. semilanceata*, which occurs in Europe and the Americas. *P. cubensis* occurs in the Americas, Asia and Australasia.

Bufotenine occurs as a secretion in cane toads including *Bufo vulgaris* and *B. viridis*. The drug also occurs in the seeds of a number of plants including *Anadenanthera peregrine* and *A. columbrina*, which are both large trees growing in South America. Other parts of the plants contain other tryptamines.

Mitragynine occurs naturally in the plant Mitragyna speciosa.

Many tryptamines may also be manufactured synthetically.

Common street names

Psilocybe mushrooms: magic mushrooms, shrooms, caps.

Bufotenine: toad, love stones.

Mitragynine: kratom.

5-Methoxy-N, N-diisopropyltryptamine: foxy, foxy methoxy.

Mechanism of action

Interaction with serotonin receptors in the brain produces alteration of auditory and visual perception.

These drugs are absorbed by the gastrointestinal tract, with an effect within 20 min of ingestion. DMT is reported to have no activity if taken orally and requires injection or coadministration with a compound to prevent first-pass metabolism.

Oral dosage of the synthetically produced tryptamines can vary from 5 mg to 100 mg, but varies significantly between similar compounds and the route of ingestion, so care is needed to avoid excessive dosage. 2 mg AMT smoked is an effective dose. Large dosages of some drugs may produce effects lasting more than 24 h. Half-lives have not been established.

Medical uses

None currently.

Legal status

Due to the varying nature of this group of compounds a generic control was applied to cover the simple tryptamines such that they are controlled by class A of the Misuse of Drugs Act 1971. Some of the newly-encountered tryptamines are not captured by that definition and the UK's ACMD recommended extension of the existing generic definition, in June 2014, to capture compounds such as AMT and 5-MeO-DALT.

Presentation and methods of administration

Powders, capsules, tablets, paper squares. Taken orally or by snorting.

Psilocybe mushrooms may be ingested as picked fresh or dried. A typical dose of fresh mushrooms would be 10–20 mushrooms but fewer for dried specimens.

Bufo toads may be licked ('toad-licking') but the dose is very variable. Many indigenous people use preparations of tryptamines in rituals, sometimes as snuffs for nasal inhalation or drinks. Again the dosage is variable.

Symptoms and signs

Acute intoxication

Physical: very varied effects can include nausea, vomiting, dizziness, and psychedelic effects including visual, temporal and auditory hallucinations.

Psychological: psychedelic effects, sometimes in waves.

Higher doses can result in disorientation, irrational behaviour, confusion, fear, delusions, paranoia and psychosis.

General/chronic

Unknown.

Driving

All likely to be incompatible with driving a motor vehicle but no known studies.

Treatment

Intoxication: nil – unless complications develop. Then supportive with monitoring of vital signs in hospital setting; intravenous benzodiazepines may be appropriate.

Further reading

Barker SA, Monti JA, Christian ST, et al. *N, N*-Dimethyltryptamine – an endogenous hallucinogen. *Int Rev Neurobiol* 1981;**22**:83–110.

Chamakura RP. Bufotenine – a hallucinogen in ancient snuff powders of South America and a drug of abuse on the streets of New York City. *Forensic Sci Rev* 1994;**6**:1–18.

Corkery JM, Durkin E, Elliott S et al. The recreational tryptamine 5-MeO-DALT (N,N-diallyl-5-methoxytryptamine): a brief review. *Progr in Neuro-psychopharmacol & Biol Psychiatry* 2011;**39**:259–262

Hasler F, Grimberg U, Benz MA, Huber T, Vollenweider FX. Acute psychological and physiological effects of psilocybin in healthy humans: a double-blind, placebo-controlled dose-effect study. *Psychopharmacology* 2004;**172**:145–56.

Meatherall R, Sharma PJ. Foxy, a designer tryptamine hallucinogen. *J Analyt Toxicol* 2003;**27**:313–17.

Passie T, Seifert J, Schneider U, Emrich HM. The pharmacology of psilocybin. *Addict Biol* 2002;**7**:357–64.

Riba J, Valle M, Urbano G, et al. Human pharmacology of ayahuasca: subjective and cardiovascular effects, monoamine metabolite excretion and pharmacokinetics. *J Pharmacol Exp Ther* 2003;**306**:73–83.

Shulgin AT, Shulgin A. *TiHKAL: The Continuation*. Berkeley, CA: Transform Press, 1997.

VOLATILE SUBSTANCES

Principal drugs

Toluene, acetone, butane, fluorocarbons, trichloroethylene, trichloroethane ethyl acetate, xylenes.

Manufacture

Laboratory/factory production.

Common street names

Gases, solvents, thinners.

Medical uses

Apart from the anaesthetic agents there are no recommended medical uses for these substances.

Mechanism of action

The solvents are rapidly absorbed through the lungs and pass into the bloodstream. They are highly lipid soluble, resulting in effects within minutes, which generally last less than an hour unless repetitive inhalation occurs.

Legal status

Widely available in shops. It is an offence to sell any intoxicating substances to a person under the age of 18, where the shopkeeper may reasonably believe that the product will be used for intoxication.

Presentation and methods of administration

A variety of compounds can be subject to misuse and the process is commonly referred to as volatile substance abuse (VSA). Compounds involved may include: solvents in adhesives (glue) such as toluene, ethyl acetate, hexane, xylenes; acetone in nail polish; fuel gases such as butane, isobutane and propane; petrol; fluorocarbons in aerosols; dry-cleaning and degreasing agents such as trichloroethylene, tetrachloroethylene, dichloromethane and trichloroethane; ozone-benign aerosol propellants such as halon; propellants in some inhalers; anaesthetic agents such as nitrous oxide or halothane.

VSA can be defined as the inhalation of such fumes in order to achieve intoxication. Vapours or gases are inhaled through the nose or mouth with the method depending on the substance misused, e.g. some products can be sniffed directly from their containers, or glue may be put in a plastic bag for inhalation ('huffing'); direct injection of lighter refills, via depression of the nozzle between the teeth, is a particularly dangerous method of ingestion.

Symptoms and signs

Acute intoxication

Physical: the solvent smell may be apparent on the breath, hands and clothing; nasal sores, burns, adhesive marks and 'glue-sniffer's rash' (perioral eczema) may be seen.

Nausea, vomiting, sneezing, coughing and diarrhoea may occur.

High doses may result in depression of the central nervous system with drowsiness, slurred speech, nystagmus, ataxia, visual disturbances and coma.

Dependence and convulsions

Sudden death is a recognised complication of solvent misuse and may occur during exposure or the post-exposure period, or result from trauma or asphyxia secondary to intoxication. Death may result from anoxia, respiratory depression, vagal inhibition and cardiac dysrhythmias. Dysrhythmias may be difficult to treat and the risk remains for several hours after inhalation. In pregnancy usage may lead to neonatal depression and there is a possibility of teratogenicity. After the acute effects wear off, there may be drowsiness and headaches with poor concentration, which may last for up to a day or so.

Psychological: euphoria with excitatory effects secondary to disinhibition (similar to alcohol but the effects occur more quickly). With increasing dosage there may be perceptual disturbances, hallucinations and delusions.

Chronic

The drugs may result in fatigue, memory impairment with poor concentration, weight loss and depression. The effects are dependent on substance abused as well as the duration and intensity of abuse.

Tolerance can develop if the misuse occurs over a prolonged period but a physical dependence syndrome is not a problem although psychological dependence may occur.

Very long-term misuse may result in liver or renal failure, liver tumours, bone marrow depression, anaemia and nervous system involvement, including cerebellar disease, dementia and peripheral neuropathy. Perioral eczema and upper respiratory tract problems may occur with chronic misuse.

Driving

Driving immediately after VSA is unlikely, although attempts may be made before the abuser's cognition and coordination have returned to normal and this would be potentially dangerous. Most road traffic offences involve people who are 'in charge' of a motor vehicle rather than actually driving.

Treatment

There are no specific treatments other than removal of the source material where possible and removal of the person from any contaminated atmosphere. Many effects are reversible on cessation of solvent misuse, except when the product is highly toxic as with leaded petrol where brain damage has occurred through lead poisoning.

Further reading

Butland BK, Field-Smith ME, Ramsey JD, et al. Twenty-five years of volatile substance abuse mortality: a national mortality surveillance programme. *Addiction* 2013;**108**:385–93.

Channer KS, Stanley S. Persistent visual hallucinations secondary to chronic solvent encephalopathy: case report and review of the literature. *J Neurol Neurosurg Psychiatry* 1983;**46**:83-86.

Flanagan RJ, Streete PJ, Ramsey JD. *Volatile Substance Abuse: Practical guidelines for analytical investigation of suspected cases and interpretation of results.* UNDCP Technical Series No.5. United Nations Drug Control Programme, Vienna, 1997.

Gunn J, Wilson J, Mackintosh AF. Butane sniffing causing ventricular fibrillation. *Lancet* 1989;**i**:617.

King MD, Day RE, Oliver RS, et al. Solvent encephalopathy. *BMJ* 1981;**283**:663–5.

Roberts MJD, McIvor RA, Adgey AAJ. Asystole following butane gas inhalation. *Br J Hosp Med* 1990;**44**:294.

Siegel E, Wason S. Sudden death caused by inhalation of butane and propane. *N Engl J Med* 1990;**323**:1638.

'Z' DRUGS

Principal drugs

Zaleplon (Sonata, Starnoc), zolpidem (Stilnoct, Ambien), zopiclone (Zimovane, Imovane), eszopiclone (Lunesta).

Common street names

Zombie, sleep-easy, zim, zimmies, zimmers.

Mechanism of action

Sedative–hypnotic drugs that depress the central nervous system.

Medical uses

These are non-benzodiazepine hypnotic drugs that act on the benzodiazepine receptors. Zaleplon is very short acting, and zopiclone and zolpidem are short acting. The half-life of zaleplon is 1 h, zolpidem 1.5–4.5 h and zopiclone 3.5–6.5 h. Zaleplon is recommended for a maximum of 2 weeks' use, and zolpidem and zopiclone for up to 4 weeks.

Legal status

These drugs are prescription-only medicines and are now all controlled under the Misuse of Drugs Act 1971 as class C drugs, with zopiclone and zaleplon having been added in June 2014.

Presentation and methods of administration

Tablets and capsules.

Symptoms and signs

Acute intoxication

Physical: sedation, with increasing doses; slurred speech, visual disturbances, loss of coordination, dysphoria, respiratory depression. All of these drugs are relatively safe in overdosage unless taken in combination with other drugs or alcohol.

Psychological: anxiolytic, impairment of memory and cognition, hallucinations, parasomnia, somnambulism.

Chronic

Sedative–hypnotic drugs may cause physical and psychological dependence and an abstinence syndrome, although such effects are reported to be rare with the 'Z' drugs unless larger than prescribed dosage is taken.

Withdrawal effects, when they occur, start within 24 h with anxiety, rebound insomnia, tremors, tachycardia and seizures having been reported.

Driving

All 'Z' drugs have the potential to impair driving ability due to their sedative effects. If taken as prescribed there are likely to be few residual effects the next morning, although patients should be warned of the possibility. Driving within a few hours of taking the drugs is likely to cause decrement of driving ability with poor concentration and coordination.

Treatment

Supportive measures are gastric lavage if recent overdose; flumazenil may be used to reverse sedation in the hospital environment.

Further reading

Drover DR. Comparative pharmacokinetics and pharmacodynamics of short-acting hypnosedatives zaleplon, zolpidem and zopiclone. *Clin Pharmacokinet* 2004;**43**:227–38.

Garnier R, Guerault E, Muzard D, et al. Acute zolpidem poisoning - analysis of 344 cases. *Clin Toxicol* 1994;**32**:391–404.

Gunja N. In the zzz zone: the effects of z drugs on human performance and driving. *J Med Toxicol* 2013;**9**:163–71.

Lader M. Zopiclone: is there any dependence and abuse potential? *J Neurol* 1997;**244**(suppl 1):S18–22.

Noble S, Langtry HD, Lamb HM. Zopiclone: an update of its pharmacology, clinical efficacy and tolerability in the treatment of insomnia. *Drugs* 1998;**55**:277–302.

Reith DM, Fountain J, McDowell R, Tilyard M. Comparison of the fatal toxicity index of zopiclone with benzodiazepines. *J Toxicol Clin Toxicol* 2003;**41**:975–80.

Terzano MG, Rossi M, Palomba V, et al. New drugs for insomnia: comparative tolerability of zopiclone, zolpidem, and zaleplon. *Drug Safety* 2003;**26**:261–82.

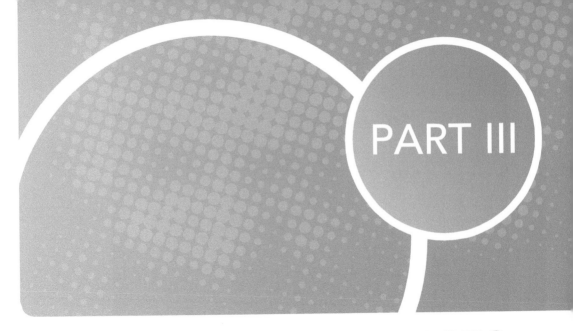

APPENDICES

APPENDIX A

Glossary

A selection of medical, technical and street terms in substance misuse (many of the names of drugs are referred to within the main text under the specific drug).

The street terms for drugs expand and change with regularity – as with those terms mentioned in relation to specific drugs, the terms below are those accepted medically, or have had regular street usage.

Please note that spellings of certain drug names vary from country to country and anyone using this book should ensure that they are making reference to the appropriate drug and name within their jurisdiction.

Abstinence – the act of refraining from the use of a substance that may lead to withdrawal syndromes such as delirium tremens or barbiturate withdrawal

Acid – LSD

Acid head – LSD user

Adam – ecstasy (MDMA)

Addict – 'a person shall be regarded as addicted to a drug only, if as a result of repeated administration he has become so dependent on the drug that he has an overpowering desire for the administration of it to be continued (and the continued administration is not required for the purpose of treating organic disease or injury)' (Misuse of Drugs [Notification of and Supply to Addicts] Regulations 1973)

ADME – refers to the processes of drug absorption (A), distribution (D), metabolism (M) and excretion (E)

Amp(s) – ampoule(s) of drugs

Angel dust – phencyclidine

Ataxia – disturbance of coordination of movement

Bag – small quantity of drugs

Barbs – barbiturate group of drugs, e.g. amylobarbital, phenobarbital

Bath salts – cathinone-type drugs

Benzos – benzodiazepine group of drugs, e.g. diazepam, nitrazepam

Billy Whizz – amphetamines

Binge – heavy episodic use of drugs (frequently alcohol, cocaine and more recently synthetic cathinones)

Bioavailability – the percentage of the administered drug that arrives unchanged in the body circulation

Biological fluid – any fluid found in the body; may include saliva, sweat, blood or urine, or vitreous humour – all of which may be used to detect drug presence

Bolivian Marching Powder – cocaine

Bong – pipe for smoking cannabis

Brown – heroin

Catecholamine – a group of hormones including adrenaline, noradrenaline and dopamine, all involved as transmitter substances in the brain

Charlie – cocaine (generally as powder)

Chasing the dragon – smoking heroin off tinfoil

Clucking – withdrawing from drugs (generally opiates)

C_{max} – maximum concentration that a drug reaches in the circulation after a single dose

CNS – central nervous system

Coke – cocaine

Crack – freebase form of cocaine; can be smoked (names include, rock, white, base)

Crystal meth – methamphetamine

Detoxification – the process whereby drug withdrawal is managed in a person dependent on alcohol or other drugs

DIC – disseminated intravascular coagulation

Dopamine – transmitter substance in brain function – a catecholamine

Dose–response effect – the likelihood and severity of an effect of a drug related to the amount of exposure to the drug

Drug – any substance, other than those required for the maintenance of normal health, which, when taken into the living organism, may modify one or more of its functions (World Health Organization)

Drug dependence (also chemical or substance dependence) – a state, psychic and sometimes also physical, resulting from the interaction between a living organism and a drug, characterised by behavioural and other responses which always include a compulsion to take the drug on a continuous or periodic basis in order to experience its psychic effects and sometimes to avoid the discomfort of its absence (World Health Organization)

Drug misuse – has been defined as any taking of a drug that harms or threatens to harm the physical and mental health or social wellbeing of an individual, other individuals or society at large, or that is illegal (Royal College of Psychiatrists, 1987)

Drug paraphernalia – items associated with drug use, e.g. syringes, needles, foil, citric acid, scales

DVLA – Driver and Vehicle Licensing Agency (in the UK)

Dysarthria – slurred speech – difficulty in articulation

E – ecstasy

ELISA – enzyme-linked immunosorbent assay – type of test used to identify drugs in biological fluids

First-pass metabolism – a process by which drugs are destroyed prior to entering the systemic circulation

Fix – injection of drugs

Flashbacks – spontaneous involuntary recurrences of drug-induced experiences

Foil – heroin may be smoked off tinfoil

Freebase – cocaine in its freebase form

Ganja – herbal cannabis

GBH – γ-hydroxybutyrate

GBL – γ-butyrolactone

Gear – illegal drugs in general

Grass – herbal cannabis

Habit (habituation) – having an addiction

Half-life – the time taken for the concentration of a drug in blood to reduce to half (assists in determining how long the effects of a drug will last)

Horse tranquilliser – ketamine

Hyperpyrexia – raised temperature

Ice – crystalline form of methamphetamine

Immunoassay – a type of biochemical test for measuring amounts of substances in biological fluids

Intravenous injection – injecting a drug directly into a vein (mainlining)

Ivory wave – cathinone-type drugs including MDPV

Joint – hand-rolled cannabis cigarette

Khat – leaves of *Catha edulis*

Kratom – hallucinogenic substance derived from the plant Mitragyna speciosa

Legal high – A substance with stimulant or mood-altering properties whose sale or use is not banned by current legislation regarding the misuse of drugs (see Aminoindanes, Indoles and Benzofurans; Phenethylamines; Piperazines; Pipradrols; Synthetic Cannabinoids; Synthetic Cathinones; Tryptamines)

Linctus – methadone

Liquid gold – amyl nitrite and related substances

Liquid ecstasy – γ-hydroxybutyrate

Liquid X – γ-hydroxybutyrate

Magic mushrooms – hallucinogenic mushrooms e.g Psilocybe

Maintenance treatment – continued use of substitution treatment as an alternative to detoxification; may be required where an individual has relapsed on several occasions after detoxification

Marijuana – herbal (leaf) cannabis

M-cat – cathinone-type drugs – often mephedrone or similar

MDMA – methylenedioxymethamphetamine (ecstasy)

Metabolite – breakdown product of the drug consumed

Meth – methamphetamine

Mexxy – methoxetamine

Meaow Meaow – cathinone-type drugs – often mephedrone or similar

Microdots – LSD

Moggies – nitrazepam (Mogadon)

Moroccan – cannabis resin

Morphine (unconjugated morphine) – as morphine sulphate, its form after administration but before metabolism in the liver; becomes conjugated morphine in the liver, mainly morphine-3-glucuronide

Mule – someone who smuggles drugs, often internally (see 'stuffer')

Munchies – excess eating stimulated by (generally) cannabis

Mushies – hallucinogenic mushrooms

MXE – methoxetamine

Nabis – cannabis

Nasal insufflation – inhaling of substances into the body via the nose

New psychoactive substance –A new narcotic or psychotropic drug, in pure form or in preparation, that is not controlled by the United Nations drug conventions, but which may pose a public health threat comparable to that posed by substances listed in these conventions (see Aminoindanes, Indoles and Benzofurans; Phenethylamines; Piperazines; Pipradrols; Synthetic Cannabinoids; Synthetic Cathinones; Tryptamines)

Nitro – amyl nitrite

NRG – cathinone-type drugs

Nystagmus – spontaneous rapid rhythmic eye movements in a side-to-side (horizontal) or up-and-down (vertical) direction

Opiates – drugs derived from the opium poppy e.g. codeine, morphine

Opioids – drugs with a treatment role in pain relief, by binding to brain opioid receptors which includes synthetic drugs e.g. methadone as well as opiates

Parenteral – generally, administration of a drug by an injection – via vein, artery, muscle or subcutaneous tissue

Pharmacodynamics – the effects of drugs on the body

Pharmacokinetics – the effects of the body on a drug

Plant food – cathinone-type drugs

Polydrug misuse – the use of more than one drug at the same time often used to titrate desired effects, ease comedown etc. Very commonly encountered; common combinations include opiates and benzodiazepines, stimulant drugs with cannabis and/or benzodiazepines it is not uncommon to find an individual addicted to opiates and benzodiazepines

Poppers – amyl nitrite and related substances

Psychoactive – any substance that affects the central nervous system and affects behaviour

Puff – herbal cannabis

Qat – khat (leaves of *Catha edulis*)

Rattling – withdrawing from drugs (generally opiates)

Recreational use (of a drug) – the use of a drug intermittently for pleasure, not associated with dependence on that drug

Reefer – cannabis cigarette

Rehabilitation – restoration of normal function

Rizla – cigarette paper – often used to roll drugs with tobacco

Rock – freebase cocaine

Roid rage – extreme aggression and violence in association with steroid use

Roofies – Rohypnol tablets

RTC – road traffic collision (formerly known as RTA – road traffic accident)

Rush – an immediate sensation of wellbeing after taking a substance

Russian Valium – phenazepam

Salt water – γ-hydroxybutyrate

Sativa – herbal cannabis

Score – to buy drugs

Script – a prescription for a drug – commonly a heroin substitute such as methadone or buprenorphine

Skin pop – the practice of injecting drugs into tissue under the skin, often leaving circular depressed scars

Skunk – potent form of cannabis

Smack – heroin

Snort – inhale drugs up nose

Snow – cocaine powder

Special K – ketamine

Speed – amphetamine

Speedball – heroin and cocaine mixed and injected (also known as snowball)

Spice – synthetic cannabinoid compounds

Spliff – hand-rolled cannabis cigarette

Stack – use of oral and injected anabolic steroids in gym culture

Stash – concealed supply of drugs

Stereotypia – persistent repetition of words or movements

Stuffer – someone who conceals large quantities of drugs in body cavities (rectum, vagina, intestine), e.g. in condoms, for purposes of smuggling

Sulphate/sulph – amphetamines

Swallower – someone who has swallowed drugs – perhaps with the intention to conceal

Synaesthesia – the experience of 'hearing colours' and 'seeing sounds'

Tab – cigarette or LSD paper

Temazzy – temazepam tablets

THC – tetrahydrocannabinol – active ingredient of cannabis

Tolerance (to a drug) – the need to increase the drug dose to get the same effect or where the same dose of a drug produces a reduced effect – occurs after repeated use of certain drugs as the body adapts

Tracks – the line(s) (often discoloured like a bruise) along a vein where impure materials (most injectable illicit drugs) have been injected. May be evident for many days or weeks

Vitamin K – ketamine

Vitreous humour – the vitreous humour is the clear gel that fills the space between the lens and the retina of the eyeball of humans

Withdrawal – the individual or cluster of symptoms and signs that are associated with the abstinence from longer-term use of some drugs (e.g. delirium tremens)

Works – needles and syringes used for injection

Wrap – small quantity of drugs

XTC – ecstasy

APPENDIX B

Clinical Institute Withdrawal Assessment of Alcohol Scale, Revised (CIWA-Ar)

Patient: _____ Date: _____ Time: _____ (24 hour clock, midnight = 00:00)

Pulse or heart rate, taken for one minute: _____ Blood pressure: _____

NAUSEA AND VOMITING – Ask "Do you feel sick to your stomach? Have you vomited?" Observation.
0 no nausea and no vomiting
1 mild nausea with no vomiting
2
3
4 intermittent nausea with dry heaves
5
6
7 constant nausea, frequent dry heaves and vomiting

TACTILE DISTURBANCES – Ask "Have you any itching, pins and needles sensations, any burning, any numbness, or do you feel bugs crawling on or under your skin?" Observation.
0 none
1 very mild itching, pins and needles, burning or numbness
2 mild itching, pins and needles, burning or numbness
3 moderate itching, pins and needles, burning or numbness
4 moderately severe hallucinations
5 severe hallucinations
6 extremely severe hallucinations
7 continuous hallucinations

TREMOR – Arms extended and fingers spread apart. Observation.
0 no tremor
1 not visible, but can be felt fingertip to fingertip
2
3
4 moderate, with patient's arms extended
5
6
7 severe, even with arms not extended

AUDITORY DISTURBANCES – Ask "Are you more aware of sounds around you? Are they harsh? Do they frighten you? Are you hearing anything that is disturbing to you? Are you hearing things you know are not there?" Observation.
0 not present
1 very mild harshness or ability to frighten
2 mild harshness or ability to frighten
3 moderate harshness or ability to frighten
4 moderately severe hallucinations
5 severe hallucinations
6 extremely severe hallucinations
7 continuous hallucinations

PAROXYSMAL SWEATS – Observation.
0 no sweat visible
1 barely perceptible sweating, palms moist
2
3
4 beads of sweat obvious on forehead
5
6
7 drenching sweats

VISUAL DISTURBANCES – Ask "Does the light appear to be too bright? Is its color different? Does it hurt your eyes? Are you seeing anything that is disturbing to you? Are you seeing things you know are not there?" Observation.
0 not present
1 very mild sensitivity
2 mild sensitivity
3 moderate sensitivity
4 moderately severe hallucinations
5 severe hallucinations
6 extremely severe hallucinations
7 continuous hallucinations

ANXIETY – Ask "Do you feel nervous?" Observation.
0 no anxiety, at ease
1 mild anxious
2
3
4 moderately anxious, or guarded, so anxiety is inferred
5
6
7 equivalent to acute panic states as seen in severe delirium or acute schizophrenic reactions

HEADACHE, FULLNESS IN HEAD – Ask "Does your head feel different? Does it feel like there is a band around your head?" Do not rate for dizziness or lightheadedness. Otherwise, rate severity.
0 not present
1 very mild
2 mild
3 moderate
4 moderately severe
5 severe
6 very severe
7 extremely severe

AGITATION – Observation.
0 normal activity
1 somewhat more than normal activity
2
3
4 moderately fidgety and restless
5
6
7 paces back and forth during most of the interview, or constantly thrashes about

ORIENTATION AND CLOUDING OF SENSORIUM – Ask "What day is this? Where are you? Who am I?"
0 oriented and can do serial additions
1 cannot do serial additions or is uncertain about date
2 disoriented for date by no more than 2 calendar days
3 disoriented for date by more than 2 calendar days
4 disoriented for place/or person

Total **CIWA-Ar** Score _____
Rater's Initials ——
Maximum Possible Score 67

The **CIWA-Ar** is not copyrighted and may be reproduced freely. This assessment for monitoring withdrawal symptoms requires approximately 5 minutes to administer. The maximum score is 67 (see instrument). Patients scoring less than 10 do not usually need additional medication for withdrawal.

Sullivan, J.T.; Sykora, K.; Schneiderman, J.; Naranjo, C.A.; and Sellers, E.M. Assessment of alcohol withdrawal: The revised Clinical Institute Withdrawal Assessment for Alcohol scale (**CIWA-Ar**). British Journal of Addiction 84:1353-1357, 1989.

APPENDIX C

Alcohol assessment questionnaires: Brief MAST, CAGE and AUDIT

The Brief MAST

		Yes	No
Questions		(Score)	
1.	Do you feel you are a normal drinker?	0	2
2.	Do friends or relatives think you're a normal drinker?	0	2
3.	Have you ever attended a meeting of Alcoholics Anonymous?	5	0
4.	Have you ever lost boyfriends/girlfriends because of drinking?	2	0
5.	Have you ever got into trouble at work because of drinking?	2	0
6.	Have you ever neglected your obligations, your family or your work for more than 2 days in a row because you were drinking?	2	0
7.	Have you ever had DTs, severe shaking, heard voices or seen things that weren't there after heavy drinking?	2	0
8.	Have you ever gone to anyone for help about your drinking?	5	0
9.	Have you ever been in hospital because of drinking?	5	0
10.	Have you ever been arrested for drunk driving or driving after drinking?	2	0

The Brief MAST is useful as a quick screening instrument to distinguish between alcohol-dependent (a score of ≥ 6) and non-alcohol-dependent individuals.

Pokorny AD, Miller BA, Kaplan HB. The Brief MAST: A shortened version of the Michigan Alcoholism Screening Test. *Am J Psychiatry* 1972;**129**:342–5.

The CAGE Questionnaire

1. Have you ever felt you should **C**ut down on your drinking?

2. Have people **A**nnoyed you by criticising your drinking?

3. Have you ever felt bad or **G**uilty about your drinking?

4. Have you ever had a drink first thing in the morning to steady your nerves, or to get rid of a hangover (**E**ye-opener)?

Two or more positive responses are a sensitive indicator of alcohol dependence.

Mayfield D, McLeod G, Hall P. The CAGE Questionnaire: Validation of a new Alcoholism Screening Instrument. *Am J Psychiatry* 1974;**131**:1121–3.

The AUDIT Questionnaire

Circle the number that comes closest to the patient's answer.

1. How often do you have a drink containing alcohol?

    (0) NEVER   (1) MONTHLY OR LESS

    (2) TWO TO FOUR TIMES A MONTH

    (3) TWO TO THREE TIMES A WEEK

    (4) FOUR OR MORE TIMES A WEEK

2. How many drinks containing alcohol do you have on a typical day when you are drinking?

    (CODE NUMBER OF STANDARD DRINKS)

    (0) 1 OR 2   (1) 3 OR 4   (2) 5 OR 6   (3) 7 OR 8   (4) 10 OR MORE

3. How often do you have six or more drinks on one occasion?

    (0) NEVER   (1) LESS THAN MONTHLY   (2) MONTHLY

    (3) WEEKLY   (4) DAILY OR ALMOST DAILY

4. How often during the last year have you found that you were not able to stop drinking once you had started?

    (0) NEVER   (1) LESS THAN MONTHLY   (2) MONTHLY

    (3) WEEKLY   (4) DAILY OR ALMOST DAILY

5. How often during the last year have you failed to do what was normally expected from you because of drinking?

    (0) NEVER   (1) LESS THAN MONTHLY   (2) MONTHLY

    (3) WEEKLY   (4) DAILY OR ALMOST DAILY

6. How often during the last year have you needed a first drink in the morning to get yourself going after a heavy drinking session?

    (0) NEVER   (1) LESS THAN MONTHLY   (2) MONTHLY

    (3) WEEKLY   (4) DAILY OR ALMOST DAILY

7. How often during the last year have you had a feeling of guilt or remorse after drinking?

    (0) NEVER   (1) LESS THAN MONTHLY   (2) MONTHLY

    (3) WEEKLY   (4) DAILY OR ALMOST DAILY

8. How often during the last year have you been unable to remember what happened the night before because you had been drinking?

(0) NEVER   (1) LESS THAN MONTHLY   (2) MONTHLY

(3) WEEKLY   (4) DAILY OR ALMOST DAILY

9. Have you or has someone else been injured as a result of your drinking?

(0) NO   (2) YES, BUT NOT IN THE LAST YEAR

(4) YES, DURING THE LAST YEAR

10. Has a relative or friend or a doctor or other health worker been concerned about your drinking or suggested you cut down?

(0) NO   (2) YES, BUT NOT IN THE LAST YEAR

(4) YES, DURING THE LAST YEAR

* In determining the response categories it has been assumed that one 'drink' contains 10 g alcohol. In countries where the alcohol content of a standard drink differs by more than 25% from 10 g, the response category should be modified accordingly.

Record sum of individual item scores here _____

A score of 8 produces the highest sensitivity; a score of ≥10 results in higher specificity. In general high scores on the first three items, in the absence of elevated scores on the remaining items, suggest hazardous alcohol use. Elevated scores on items 4–6 imply the emergence of alcohol dependence. High scores on the remaining items suggest harmful alcohol use.

Babor TF, Ramon de la Fuente J, Saunders J, Grant M. *AUDIT The Alcohol Use Disorders Identification Test: Guidelines for use in Primary Health Care.* Geneva: World Health Organization, 1992.

APPENDIX D

Clinical Opiate Withdrawal Scale

Patient's Name:_____

Date and Time:_____/_____/_____

Resting Pulse Rate:_____beats/minute
Measured after patient is sitting or lying for one minute
  0 pulse rate 80 or below
  1 pulse rate 81–100
  2 pulse rate 101–120
  4 pulse rate greater than 120

Sweating: *Over past 1/2 hour not accounted for by room temperature or patient activity*
  0 no report of chills or flushing
  1 subjective report of chills or flushing
  2 flushed or observable moistness on face
  3 beads of sweat on brow or face
  4 sweat streaming off face

Restlessness: *Observation during assessment*
  0 able to sit still
  1 reports difficulty sitting still, but is able to do so
  3 frequent shifting or extraneous movements of legs/arms
  5 unable to sit still for more than a few seconds

Pupil size:
  0 pupils pinned or normal size for room light
  1 pupils possibly larger than normal for room light
  2 pupils moderately dilated
  5 pupils so dilated that only the rim of the iris is visible

Bone or Joint aches: *If patient was having pain previously, only the additional component attributed to opiates withdrawal is scored*
  0 not present
  1 mild diffuse discomfort
  2 patient reports severe diffuse aching of joints/muscles
  4 patient is rubbing joints or muscles and is unable to sit still because of discomfort

Runny nose or tearing: *Not accounted for by cold symptoms or allergies*
  0 not present
  1 nasal stuffiness or unusually moist eyes
  2 nose running or tearing
  4 nose constantly running or tears streaming down cheeks

GI Upset: *Over last 1/2 hour*
  0 no GI symptoms
  1 stomach cramps
  2 nausea or loose stool
  3 vomiting or diarrhea
  5 Multiple episodes of diarrhea or vomiting

Tremor: *Observation of outstretched hands*
  0 no tremor
  1 tremor can be felt, but not observed
  2 slight tremor observable
  4 gross tremor or muscle twitching

Yawning: *Observation during assessment*
  0 no yawning
  1 yawning once or twice during assessment
  2 yawning three or more times during assessment
  4 yawning several times/minute

Anxiety or Irritability:
  0 none
  1 patient reports increasing irritability or anxiousness
  2 patient obviously irritable or anxious
  4 patient so irritable or anxious that participation in the assessment is difficult

Gooseflesh skin:
  0 skin is smooth
  3 piloerection of skin can be felt or hair standing up on arms
  5 prominent piloerection

Total score:_____
The total score is the sum of all 11 items
(5–12 = mild   13–24 = moderate   25–36 = moderately severe   >36 = severe withdrawal)

Initials of person completing assessment:_____

Reference: California Society of Addiction Medicine

APPENDIX E

Further Reading and Resources

Advisory Council on the Misuse of Drugs (ACMD). Available from: www.homeoffice.gov.uk/agencies-public-bodies/acmd/ (accessed 3 June 2013).

Canadian Centre on Substance Abuse. *Harm Reduction: Concepts and Practice: A Policy Discussion Paper*. Canadian Centre on Substance Abuse (CCSA), National Working Group on Policy, 1996.

Chief Medical Officer. *Medical Care of Suspected Internal Drug traffickers – Independent Report of the Chief Medical Officer's Expert Group, 25 January 2013*. Available from: https://www.gov.uk/government/publications/report-on-the-care-of-suspected-internal-drug-traffickers (accessed 5 June 2013).

Department of Health. *A summary of the health harms of drugs*, 2011. Available from: www.dh.gov.uk/en/Publicationsandstatistics/Publications/PublicationsPolicyAndGuidance/DH_129624 (accessed 5 June 2013).

European Monitoring Centre for Drugs and Drug Addiction (EMCDDA). Available from: www.emcdda.europa.eu (accessed 5 June 2013).

European Workplace Drug Testing Society (EWDTS). *Guidelines for Legally Defensible Workplace Drug Testing Specimen Collection Procedures*. Available from: www.ewdts.org/data/uploads/documents/specimen-collection-guidelines_oct11.pdf (accessed 5 June 2013).

Faculty of Forensic and Legal Medicine. *Guidelines for Doctors Asked to Perform Intimate Body Searches*. London: Royal College of Physicians, 2007. Available from: www.fflm.ac.uk (Accessed 5 June 2013).

Faculty of Forensic and Legal Medicine. *Taking Blood Specimens from Incapacitated Drivers*. London: Royal College of Physicians, 2010. Available from: www.fflm.ac.uk (accessed 5 June 2013).

Faculty of Forensic and Legal Medicine. *Substance Misuse Detainees in Police Custody. Guidelines for clinical management*. London: Royal College of Physicians, 2011. Available from: www.fflm.ac.uk (accessed 5 June 2013).

Ghodse H, Corkery J, Claridge H, Goodair C, Schifano F. *Drug-related deaths in the UK (January–December 2011). Annual Report 2012*. National Programme on Substance Abuse Deaths (*np*-SAD), International Centre for Drug Policy (ICDP), St George's, University of London, UK. Available from: www.sgul.ac.uk/research/projects/icdp/our-work-programmes/substance-abuse-deaths (accessed 6 June 2013).

Health Protection Agency. Available from: www.hpa.org.uk/Publications/InfectiousDiseases/BloodBorneInfections/ShootingUp/1211Shootingup2012 (accessed 5 June 2013).

Lenton S, Single E. The definition of harm reduction. *Drug Alcohol Rev* 1998;**17**:213–20.

Newcombe R. The reduction of drug-related harm: a conceptual framework for theory, practice and research. In: O'Hare PA, Newcombe R, Mathews A, et al. (eds), *The Reduction of Drug-Related Harm*. London: Routledge, 1992.

Parrot AC. Recreational Ecstasy/MDMA, the serotonin syndrome, and serotonergic neurotoxicity. *Pharmacol Biochem Behav* 2002;**71**:837–44.

UK Home Office. www.gov.uk/government/announcements

United Nations Office on Drugs and Crime. *Guidelines for the Forensic Analysis of Drugs Facilitating Sexual Assault and Other Criminal Acts*, 2011. Available from: www.unodc.org/documents/scientific/forensic_analys_of_drugs_facilitating_sexual_assault_and_other_criminal_acts.pdf (accessed 5 June 2013).

US Food and Drug Administration. FDA Public Health Advisory. *Combined Use of 5-Hydroxytryptamine Receptor Agonists (Triptans), Selective Serotonin Reuptake Inhibitors (SSRIs) or Selective Serotonin/Norepinephrine Reuptake Inhibitors (SNRIs) May Result in Life-threatening Serotonin Syndrome.* Rockville, MD: Center for Drug Evaluation and Research, 2006.

Vilke G, Payne-James JJ, Karch SB. Excited delirium syndrome: redefining an old diagnosis. *J Forensic Legal Med* 2012;**19**:7–11.

INDEX